Ketogenic Bread

70+ Low-Carb Recipes for Ketogenic Bread, Buns, Crackers, and More!

Table of Contents

Introduction

Congratulations on purchasing *Ketogenic Bread: Low Carb Recipes for Ketogenic Bread, Buns, Crackers, and More!* And thank you for doing so. Getting started with the Keto diet can be somewhat intimidating for beginners. Aside from the stress that goes along with going on any diet, there is always the common question of what to eat while maintaining a satisfied pallet. A common deterrent for people starting the Keto diet is the issue of having to give up bread entirely. Well, with the help of this book you won't have to worry about crossing that obstinate obstacle.

The following chapters will discuss a variety of different types of ways to enjoy the taste and familiarity of bread while on the going keto. From bread loaves to muffins, bagels, and much more, you will be able to find a variety of delectable recipes to choose from while you make the transition into the Keto lifestyle. You can use these as substitutes for regular bread, as snacks, or even a full meal on their own!

Before diving into the recipes, we will cover what the Ketogenic diet is, basic ideas behind the science and lifestyle, as well as give a rundown on the premise that the diet has been founded upon; Ketosis. When perusing through the recipes themselves, there will be listed the nutritional data to make sure everything is low in calories, carbohydrates, and everything else you need to stay on track to reach your dieting goals. Another thing you will discover when looking over the recipes is that many of the ingredients in this book are of the utmost healthy variety. A trip to your local health food store is recommended, not just for this book, but to keep the goals of your dieting in eyesight no matter what else is going on.

There are plenty of books on this subject on the market, thanks again for choosing this one.! Every effort was made to ensure it is full of as much useful information as possible, please enjoy!

Chapter 1: What is Ketosis?

Chances are that you have heard of the ketogenic diet before. Its origins can be traced back to 1921. During that year, Rollin Woodyatt did some research with the aim of discovering links between people's diets and diabetes. The results went much further than anyone at the time could have imagined.

What he discovered was 3 water-soluble compounds (hydroxybutyrate, acetone, and acetoacetate) that are collectively known as the ketone bodies. While this discovery was first used to help alleviate epileptic symptoms in children, it would also lead the way to understand how the human body uses these ketone bodies, and thus, later lead to the keto diet.

The basic premise of the keto diet can come across as confusing, but it does not have to be. Granted, the science behind it is a science and thus is bogged down by many technical complications, but you don't have to be a full-blown dietician to understand the major pillars of what makes up the ketogenic diet.

The keto (key-toe) diet is low in carbohydrates, moderate in protein, and high in fat. Right away when someone hears that a tenant of the keto diet is that its high in fat, many people would turn away. The thing that must be understood is that the human body will either use ketones or glucose to provide energy. These two different ways of fueling the body have gained popular labels that you may have heard getting tossed around quite often. When someone's diet consists of mostly carbohydrates, they are often referred to as being a "sugar burning machine." Yet, when someone's diet does not consist of mostly carbohydrates, they are often referred to as being a "fat burning machine." The calories we consume are not the villains they have been made out to be. It is what our bodies convert the calories into that matters.

In today's modern society most people are sugar-burning machines. They receive their calories from glucose. Please understand that glucose is sugar, and when intaking carbs, those carbs will be converted into glucose. The catch is that the human body can only store so much glucose and whatever excess glucose it has acquired will be converted into body fat that does not get used. Glucose is easy for the body to convert to energy and the body will select to use that instead of using fat as fuel. Then that fat will just sit there in all the places you don't want it to be. If this goes on for several years, then the pounds can add up to a substantial amount.

Although it would be nice to point a finger at the human physiological system and chastise it, we can't blame the body for being confused on what we want it to use for energy. If it is regularly receiving more glucose then fat, then, of course, it is going to hold onto the fat (since it does not know when it will receive more of it) and select to burn and utilize the glucose (since there is a constant stream of carbs being poured into it). The human body is very good at managing resources and is simply saving less of one resource (fat) and using more of another, more abundant, resource (glucose). This is why, when someone intakes more glucose than fat, then they will often have cravings to reach for a candy bar or bag of chips.

The human body can become far too accustomed to selecting glucose as its main energy resource, and it will begin to panic when there is not enough glucose to use. Then it will issue a command to fill up on more glucose. For many people, reaching for those chips or candy bars is the quickest way to pump more glucose into the system and alleviate the body's panics and cravings. After eating the candy bar or chips, the body will burn the glucose as it has been trained to do, and leave the extra fat sitting there, as it has also been trained to do.

But it doesn't have to be that way. The body can be retrained to work the other way and turn into a fat-burning machine instead of a sugar-burner.

What if you did not have so many carbs in your diet? Well, then your body would have to recognize that there has a been a shift in its available resources and make the proper switch. It would start to burn off the excess fat already in the body and use that as its main energy source instead of glucose. This also means that it would be storing less fat (since it would also be using that new fat for energy as well). Since the body would be turning newly consumed fats into energy, and, also turning the fats that have already been stored away into energy- weight loss must happen. Not only must it happen, but it must continue to happen as well. The fat that has previously been stored away will burn off and convert into energy, which will result in weight loss. While this is happening, simultaneously the newly consumed fats will also convert into energy and not into excess body fat, which means that the lost weight will not have a chance to return and anchor itself down.

Have you ever heard of the fact that the human body can last several weeks without food but only a few days without water? Why would that be? The answer is because most people have enough fat stored away to last them for some time and (if placed in such a harrowing situation) the body would begin to burn away the stored fat for survival. Now, in this book, we are talking about dieting and cooking, not being stranded on a desert island. Please don't think that such a perilous trial awaits you. With proper recipes and knowledge in hand, you certainly won't have to starve yourself. Well, you will have to starve yourself of carbohydrates, but more on that later.

When the human body is in this state of using fat as its main energy source instead of glucose, it will enter a metabolic phase known as "Ketosis." Getting the body into ketosis (and maintaining it) is the goal of going on a ketogenic diet. When you hear the phrase "fat-burning machine," know that ketosis is what is being specifically referred to. When your body has entered the state of ketosis, it has successfully been retrained to recognize fat as its main resource for fuel and will no longer shy away from burning it off. Again, the human body is very good at resource management, and all it really needs to know is what resource it has more available to use.

But how is this retraining of the body accomplished? How can we get our bodies to make the switch into ketosis and become a fat-burning machine? How do we get the body to recognize which resource is the one we want it to use for energy and burn away? How do we get the body into ketosis, and what exactly is going on when we have entered the ketogenic state?

Switch the main resources used for fuel, and the machine will operate differently. If you take in more fat then carbs, the body will naturally start to enter ketosis. Lowering the carbs and increasing the fat is the major trick to reaching this. If there is any starving going on when you are trying to enter ketosis, it is the starvation of carbohydrates mentioned earlier. However, you do not need to eliminate carbs entirely to get your body into ketosis. What you do need to do is eat a diet that is low in carbs, higher in fat, and moderate in protein. Doing so will set up the foundations to switch your body from using fat instead of glucose as its main energy resource. So, you see that when hearing of a diet that is high in fat, there is really no reason to turn away from it

When the body is in ketosis, it will produce the ketones that were mentioned previously. Ketones are the chemical compounds that fat can be converted into to be used for energy. Knowing this, it is easy to understand that dropping the unwanted pounds is going to be a result of having ketones in the body, but are there any other benefits?

Having ketones in the body can also help improve the overall blood flow going on in the human system. This can help balance out blood sugar, improve oxygen capacity, increase energy levels, help assist in athletic performance, and be conducive to mental clarity. If that wasn't enough, they could also help improve generating healthy masses of muscles, act as mood stabilizers (in type 2 bipolar disorder), help reduce migraines, and improve cholesterol levels. What's more, ketones have been known to help prevent metabolic syndrome management, strokes, and certain cardiovascular diseases. Among some members of the medical field, increasing ketone levels is recommended to stave off the effects of Parkinson's disease, Alzheimer's, multiple sclerosis, and other maladies. Knowing this, is there any wonder why some people refer to ketones as a "super-fuel"?

With so many benefits related to having ketones in the body, why isn't everyone going the keto way and diving into ketosis yet? Different people will provide different answers to that, but a common detractor is that people have trouble giving up the carbs. Lowering intake of sugar is difficult enough for some, but when trying to lower carbs in general, many people hit a brick wall when they realize that one thing they need to stop consuming is bread.

That is exactly why this book was constructed so anyone who is trying to move into the keto lifestyle will find an easier transition knowing that they can replace their old recipes and ideas of bread for brand new ones! Yes, the old way you used to view bread has to go, but many if not all of your old favorite ways to eat bread do not. You can still have toast with your bacon and eggs, still, eat your burger with a bun, and don't have to say goodbye to bagels or sandwiches. You just need to learn how to replace the old regular bread (and carbs) with new recipes (and ketones). Retraining the body to select a better fuel, increase efficacy, and lose the extra pounds has never tasted or felt so good before.

Chapter 2: Clearing up the Keto Controversy

Before moving any further, it should be stated clearly that this book is not designed to replace your doctor and is not a medical manual. If your doctor has prescribed that you go on a ketogenic diet for whatever reason, then you should follow their orders at all times. Don't be afraid to doublecheck with them on anything that you may lack clarity on. First, understand why they placed you on a ketogenic diet, then take it from there.

Believe it or not, your body has probably entered a state of ketosis before. Chances are that when it did, it was only the starting stages and was so mild that you just didn't notice any difference. Then, you may have filled up on carbs again and stopped the body from getting used to being ketosis and adapting to it. If you have ever fasted, just missed a meal or two, exercised for an hour or more, or simply slept in for a long time (we all have done this at least a few times) then you probably began the process of ketosis but didn't know it, and thus, didn't continue to let the ketones work their fat obliterating magic.

The keto diet has differing opinions on how it is done. Just about everyone will agree that it is high in fat, moderate in protein, and lower in carbs. Most would also agree on what foods are allowed and which are not. After that, the debates begin. We are not going to cover all of that here as it would take another book to entirely cover all of the differing points of view on the keto diet. Yet, there are at least a few things you should know and expect when transitioning from a normal carb filled diet into the keto lifestyle.

First off, cement the word *lifestyle* into your brain. Sorry to be harsh but dieting just will not work for the long-term if you do not adapt to everything that goes along with it. Along with watching what you eat and replacing your old ideas of bread with a new way of viewing and eating it, regular exercise should become a habit to ingrain into your weekly routines. At the very least, if you don't already, add some light cardio into your schedule a few days a week. When combining exercise with ketosis, your body may be confused at first but will very quickly start showing off results and thanking you whole heartily.

Remember that for the keto diet to work long-term you need to keep your body in the state of ketosis more than it is not. This is an issue that many people get confused with and sometimes overdue or overlook some things. If you have gotten your body into ketosis, and then for whatever reason, you fall out of ketosis for only a few hours, that is not the end of the road. Many people will panic when checking their ketone levels and seeing them minutely dip. Panicking won't help get those levels back to where you want them to be, commitment will. Some of the controversy surrounding the ketogenic diet is nothing more than placing too much emphasis on the small and not the whole. As long as you are sticking with it, seeing, and feeling the results of being in ketosis more then you are not, then there is nothing to worry about. Once again, being in ketosis is a lifestyle change and retraining of how the body works. With dieting and everything else in life, if you really want long-term results, then a commitment be made.

To help alleviate some of the panic and confusion that comes along when someone is staring at the ketogenic diet, remember these rules:

- Consume less than 100 carbs a day. 100 carbs a day is pushing it, so consider that the absolute maximum. To go the extra mile in ensuring that ketosis will happen and keeps happening, aim for no more than 50 carbs a day.

- Consume more dietary fat than carbs. Most of your calories should come from fat.

- There are good fats and bad fats. To keep it simple, saturated fats are bad. Monosaturated fats are good. The ingredients in this book are loaded with monosaturated fats.

- Remember these ratios: 5-10% of carbohydrates. 15-30% of protein. 60-75% fat. Keep those numbers in mind for your daily caloric consumption and meal planning.

- Do some research to find out which foods are and are not allowed on the keto diet. This book is only designed to cover bread replacements (no grains on keto). However, many of the foods that are allowed when aiming for ketosis (wild meats, leafy green veggies, eggs, many others) we are used to eating along with bread. If you are slapping the wrong type of meat in-between the right kind of bread though, ketosis may be stalled.

- It is worth mentioning again. Follow your doctor's orders. This is not a medical book and you, above everyone else, are responsible for your own health.

There are just a few more tidbits of information you should know before diving into the recipes.

The first has already been mentioned earlier, and it is the concept of fasting. Fasting is the most natural way to enter a state of ketosis. When fasting, it is ketosis that keeps the body alive. Different people have different reasons for fasting, and the benefits of doing so are well documented. It is not something most people would consider very fun though, and when trying to add exercise into your life while fasting your body may run into a state of confliction. When going on the keto diet, you do not need to fast and can still receive many of the benefits from doing so without throwing your body into a state of confusion. Since ketosis is a natural physiological process, we can combine it with our modern knowledge of nutrition and get the best of both worlds.

When starting the keto diet, most people will see results so quickly that they will have a hard time believing what they see in the mirror. The reason for this is the quick reduction of water weight. When entering ketosis, water weight will be the first to go. Keep in mind that to garner the maximum benefits of going on a keto diet, you need to keep your body in ketosis much more then it is not. Losing the water weight will get you off to a good start, but that is only the beginning. The goal is to turn your body into a fat-burning machine. You have to lose the water weight first before obliterating the fat, and you will if you stick with it.

Something that those who don't support the keto diet like to warn people about is known as the "keto flu." This is a slightly unfair label to attach to the diet but is not entirely wrong either. When you make sudden changes in the resources your body uses, some disruption is to be expected. The body is used to operating in a certain manner, relying upon the resource of glucose. Keep in mind that while the body is being retrained to not depend upon carbs that there will be a period of withdrawal. This stage won't last long though, and there a few things you can do to minimize its effects or maybe even circumvent it all together.

- Start slow. Lower your carb intake a little bit at a time to make the transition smoother.

- Make sure that you are giving the body the correct amount of fuel by eating enough fats.

- Water. Drink plenty of water to stay hydrated.

If you find that you have trouble falling asleep, feel slight stomach pains, lack concentration, become irritable, nauseous, or feel muscles soars, then you have been bitten by the keto flu. There may also be an overall lack of energy at first (but when your body gets used to being in ketosis you will feel surges of abundant energy). First off, understand that again, dieting is a lifestyle change and sticking with the diet and keeping your goals in eyesight will have better long-term results than the short-term discomforts and bothers. If you do fall victim to the keto flu though, there are some steps you can take to get over it fairly quickly.

- Water. Same as when trying to avoid the flu. Stay hydrated with plenty of water.

- Exercise. Already mentioned before but worth hammering in. A little bit of light cardio a few times a week can go a very long way. It should be made clear though, do not overdo the exercise when first going on a keto diet. As time goes on you can increase your levels and length of exercise, but just start with 30 minutes of cardio a few times during the week. If you have already been bitten by the keto flu bug, keep the exercise light and gentle. Even a walk around your neighborhood is enough to do the trick.

- Be sure that you are taking in enough electrolytes. This can easily be accomplished by consuming salts and bone broths. Drinking some Gatorade may also help, but do not mistake it as a replacement for water.

The keto flu generally only lasts about 1 week when you are first starting out. Although some have reported that it may last for the entirety of the first month when moving from a normal diet into a ketogenic one. Follow the guidelines above to prevent this from happening.

Another complaint some detractors to the keto diet claim is that it will cause constipation. This can result from the same reasons as the keto flu, the shift going on in the body when retraining it to recognize one resource over another. Of course, no one wants to have to deal with constipation, and there are ways to avoid that from happening as well.

- Water. Are you getting the point yet how important it is to stay hydrated?
- Drink tea to settle the stomach.
- Keep up a regular feeding schedule, so your body has fewer things to be confused about.
- Consume vegetables that are fibrous.
- Try a magnesium supplement.
- Be moderate with consumption of nuts.
- Consume Coconut oil, Chia seeds, and Flaxseeds (all of which you will find within the recipes in this book).

As a final note, when transitioning into ketosis, there may be spikes to desire more carbs. Also, some people just don't think they have a pallet that enjoys eating many keto friendly foods and recipes. Guess what, those cravings will pass after your body gets used to being in ketosis, and the pallet will begin to enjoy the foods that it previously did not. The taste buds are a part of the body too, and retraining the body is what being in ketosis is all about.

Just remember that for any diet to work long-term, a change of lifestyle and commitment is required. When done correctly, with the right selection of foods and recipes, being in ketosis will change your body and life for the better.

Chapter 3: A Brief Note on The Ingredients

While reading this book and looking over the recipes, you may come across several ingredients that may be unfamiliar to you. This is common for people who are new to the keto diet (and even a few of the old hands may discover something new while giving this book a look over). Remember that the goal of this book is to replace your old ideas of bread with a new one, and something that is bound to happen while making the switch from a normal diet to the keto way is baking with ingredients that you may not have previously been familiar with. To help you along the way of grasping how to bake keto replacement bread, a short explanation of some of the less well-known ingredients is listed in this chapter.

Butter- Everyone knows what butter is. When going keto though, the question of what type of butter to use may arise and cause some confusion. It's really not that hard to figure out and does not need to be so mysterious. When reading this book and seeing the word butter pop up for an ingredient, know that what is intended is grass-fed butter.

Grass-fed butter has many health benefits over grain-fed butter. It contains more Omega-3 fatty acids and also has more of the vitamin K2. Both of these have major health benefits and that alone trumps grass-fed butter over grain-fed. There is also a specific fatty acid known as CLA (conjugated linoleic acid), and grass-fed butter has 5 times more of the amount inside of it then grain-fed butter. As you can see from reading this, if the cows we consume eat healthier, then we eat healthier as well.

Another ingredient that commonly pops up when looking into keto circles is called Ghee. Ghee is not listed for any of the recipes in this book. However, any swapping out of butter for Ghee would not cause a problem as they are very similar. For those of you who are avoiding or trying to eliminate lactose from your diet, you can replace the butter for Ghee without worry.

Salts- Salt is a common staple for most people who go on a keto diet. When the body goes into ketosis, and when going on a low carb diet in general, the blood sodium levels may drop. To counteract this adding salt to your food and recipes is recommended.

But what types of salt to use? The three types of salt you will see listed in this book are the following: salt (regular), pink Himalayan salt, and sea salt. Although the specific types that are listed in each recipe are recommended, they can be swapped out for each other without worry.

Sweeteners- Sugar has no place on a keto diet. If there is an enemy in the world of keto, sugar shelters the enemy, waiting to strike against all you have been working towards. That doesn't mean that you have to retire the sweet tooth forever though. Many of the recipes in this book will require a touch of sweetness, and as such, non-sugar-based substitutes will be listed. When it comes to these types of sweeteners, there are many different options to choose from but to make things a little easier only two are listed in this book. They are Stevia and erythritol. Both of these are common in the keto world. You may replace one for the other if you desire.

Contrary to what was already said, erythritol does contain sugar, but will not raise blood sugar levels and is safe for people with diabetes. The sugar is in there, somewhere, but has been chained down and unable to strike from the confines of its prison.

Besides adding a touch of sweet to the world of baking, erythritol serves another purpose. It can act as a leveling agent the same way that baking soda does. Leveling agents are required for certain recipes as they can make sure that everything rises and mixes correctly.

For Stevia, it is good to know that it comes in a liquid and powdered form. It can also, if desired, be found in leaf form but the stevia listed in this book will primarily be considered the powdered form with the liquid one appearing for certain recipes.

One last thing to mention about sugar when baking, often times sugar will be "cooked out" of food when the dish is done baking. Again, sugar has no place in the world of keto, and this book does not contain any recipes that will insert sugar into your body.

Cream of tartar- This can act as another leveling agent when baking. Aside from that, it contains another benefit when going keto. Some people may run into lowering their potassium a bit too much when starting the keto diet. Cream of tartar can act as a potassium supplement to help avoid those levels from dropping too low.

Xanthan Gum- This one helps when baking because it can assist in holding and combining different ingredients together. It also acts as a substitute for gluten (another enemy for those who are going on a keto diet). Something to take note of here though is that there are some xanthan gums that do have gluten in them. So, when shopping for xanthan gum make sure you purchase a gluten free one.

Psyllium Husk Powder- Psyllium husk can also act as a replacement for gluten and wheat, but it is worth mentioning that whenever it is seen popping up in this book that it will specifically be the powder form that is intended to be used. Whole psyllium husk is not recommended for these recipes as that has been known to cause some unwanted side effects. Don't use whole psyllium husk, stick to the powder.

Another note about the psyllium husk powder is that it can alter the color of bread to a purple shade. There is nothing to fear here as the bread will still be edible and tasty. However, most people may not want their bread to be purple. There is a very easy fix for this, and it is listed along with most of the instructions used for baking but is also stated here for clarification. If using psyllium husk powder, use an egg wash to brush the bread before baking. Doing so will prevent the color from turning purple and will give the bread a nice and shiny, professional looking, gleam.

Soy Protein Isolate- This one does not appear in this book too often, but you will still see it from time to time. It is used to help moderate the protein levels. Many recipes floating around out there will call for Whey protein isolate. The reason that soy is used in this book is because if protein levels go too high then your body may exit ketosis. There are many variables on this, as everyone's body is different. For some people there may not be a problem with using the whey protein isolate, but the soy option has been selected for this book to avoid spiking protein levels for those that the whey would not benefit. If you so desire, then go ahead and use the Whey protein isolate.

Parchment paper- No, you don't eat this. Please don't try to eat this. It will pop up often for several times in the recipes, and if you are new to cooking, then a brief explanation of how to use it is explained below for you.

Typically speaking many chefs will place parchment paper on a baking sheet then the dough to be baked atop the parchment paper, then place another sheet of parchment paper on top of the dough. With the dough sandwiched between two sheets of parchment paper, it will then be smoothed with a person's hand or rolling pin. You don't have to do it that way, but it is recommended and is also what the professionals do. The second sheet of parchment paper, the one on top, should be removed before baking.

Blenders and Food Processors- These tools are more or less the same thing. The only reason they are noted here is in case you are confused by the word "pulse." Some of these devices do not have that option, while others do. Just be aware that "pulse" is the fastest speed, and you should be fine.

Serving sizes- Many of the recipes can fluctuate on what the serving sizes actually are. A loaf of bread may say that it makes 16 servings, but it can't be guaranteed that everyone will cut the same sized slice. For this reason, the serving sizes are recommended portions but expect some variability.

Measurements- This final note is only for people who are brand new to cooking just so no one gets confused. Almost all the measurements in this book are teaspoons (tsp), tablespoons (Tbsp), and cups. This is done for consistency. Keep in mind that the numbers for the measurements are considered universal; 0.25 for a tsp or Tbsp is the literal amount listed. 0.25 cups are one-fourth of a cup, 0.50 is one half of a cup, and so on.

Now that all that is out of the way you can head on over to the kitchen and get stated reimagining your old concepts of bread and baked goods for a new and better way.

Chapter 4: Bread Loaves – the Keto Way

One of the first things to get started on when moving into a Keto lifestyle is replacing your old understanding of bread with a new and healthier one. Here are some Keto bread replacements to get you started!

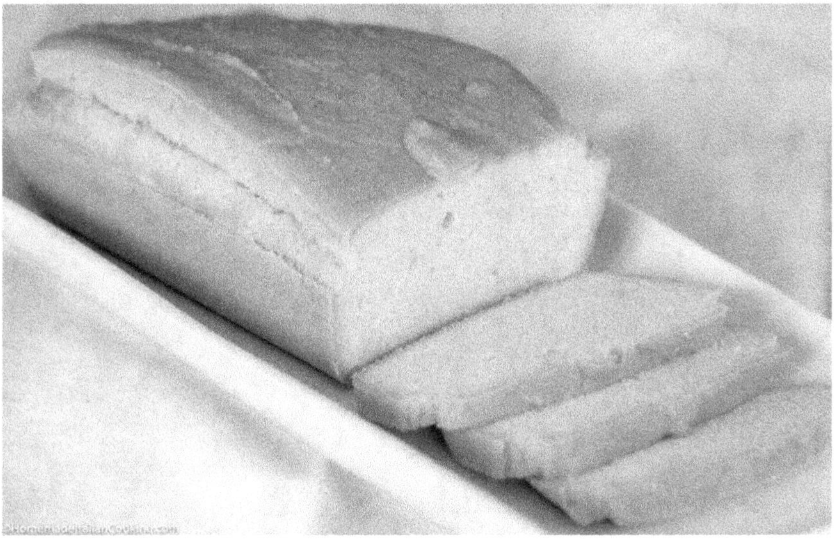

Easy Keto Bread

This recipe takes about 80 minutes to prepare and bake and makes 18 servings.

- Calories: 82
- Carbs: 3 grams
- Fat:7 grams
- Fiber: 2 grams
- Protein: 4 grams

What to Use

- 12 large egg whites
- 0.75 cups of butter (melted)
- 0.25 tsp of sea salt
- 2 tsp of baking powder
- 0.25 cups of coconut flour
- 1 cup of almond flour
- 0.25 tsp of xanthan gum

Baking Instructions

- Preheat oven to 325F. While that is warming up go and grab a baking pan and line it with parchment paper. Also, make sure to melt the butter.

- Go get a food processor and place inside it the coconut flour, baking powder, sea salt, and xanthan gum. Pulse everything until they combine well.

- Add the melted butter into the mix. Pulse for about 5 seconds until it combines.

- Go get a large bowl and toss in all the egg whites. Use a hand mixer to beat the eggs.

- Add half of the contents from the bowl of egg whites into the food processor. Pulse for only a few seconds until it begins to combine.

- Then pour the contents of the food processor back into the large bowl with remaining egg whites. Gently fold everything in and try not to deflate the egg whites. You do not need to do any stirring here.

- Transfer the batter into the baking pan.

- Bake for 40 minutes. Stop baking for a moment to top the pan with an aluminum foil dome. Then bake for another 30 minutes.

Low Carb Keto Bread

This recipe takes about 55 minutes to prepare and bake and makes 10 servings.

- Calories: 139
- Carbs: 3 grams
- Fat: 12 grams
- Fiber: 1 gram
- Protein: 4 grams

What to Use

- 3 tsp of baking powder
- 0.50 tsp of sea salt
- 2 Tbsp of coconut oil
- 0.50 cup of butter
- 2 cups of almond meal
- 1 tsp of psyllium husk powder
- 0.50 cups of butter
- 7 large eggs

Baking Instructions

- Preheat oven to 350F. While it is warming up, melt the butter and separately melt the coconut oil. Do not melt them together. Also, grab a baking pan while you are at it and grease it up.

- Put the eggs in a large bowl. Use a hand mixer to mix them for three minutes.
- And the coconut oil (make sure it is melted). Mix it with the eggs for about one minute.
- Mix in the butter (make sure that is melted too) and mix it with the eggs and coconut oil for another minute.
- Place the salt, baking powder, psyllium husks powder and almond meal into the bowl. Mix them together till they begin to from together.
- Transfer the dough into the loaf pan.
- Bake for 50 minutes. Let cool for 10.

Keto Protein Bread

This recipe takes about 40 minutes to prepare and bake and makes 20 servings.

- Calories: 50
- Carbs: 3 grams
- Fat: 3 grams
- Fiber: 2 grams
- Protein: 5 grams

What to Use

- 1 Tbsp of apple cider vinegar
- 2 tsp of baking powder
- 0.25 tsp of pink Himalayan salt
- 1 tsp of psyllium husk powder
- 3 large eggs
- 0.50 cups of cream cheese
- 0.25 cups of soy protein isolate
- 0.25 tsp of coconut oil

Baking Instructions

- Preheat oven to 320F. While that is warming up go and grab a baking pan and grease it up.

- Grab a large bowl and place inside it the soy protein isolate, Himalayan salt, baking powder, and psyllium husk powder. Whisk everything together until it blends together.

- Go grab a medium bowl and place inside it the cream cheese. Use a whisk to soften the cream cheese.

- While softening the cream cheese, add the eggs, but only do so one at a time. In between the adding of the eggs, keep whisking.

- Add the coconut oil to the bowl of cream cheese and eggs. Whisk everything, so it combines with well.

- Pour the bowl of coconut oil, cream cheese, and eggs into the bowl of soy, salt, and all their friends. Whisk everything until they combine and form together well.

- Add in the apple cider vinegar. Whisk it to combine with everything.

- Let everything settle for 5 minutes.

- Transfer the batter into the baking pan.

- Bake for 35 minutes.

Keto Low Carb Protein Seeded Bread

This recipe takes about 40 minutes to prepare and bake and makes 16 servings.

- Calories: 58
- Carbs: 2.5 grams
- Fat: 4 grams
- Fiber: 4 grams
- Protein: 4.5 grams

What to Use

- 1 Tbsp of apple cider vinegar
- 3 Tbsp of chia and flaxseed mixture
- 2 tsp of baking powder
- 0.16 tsp of pink Himalayan salt
- 1 tsp of psyllium husk powder
- 0.75 cups of soy protein isolate
- 1 cup of cream cheese
- 3 large eggs

Baking Instructions

- Preheat oven to 300F. While that is warming up grab a baking pan and grease it up.

- Grab a large bowl and place inside the baking powder, soy protein isolate, psyllium husk powder, and salt. Whisk everything together until it combines well.

- Go grab a medium bowl and place inside it the cream cheese. Use a whisk to soften the cream cheese.

- While softening the cream cheese, add the eggs, but only do so one at a time. In between the adding of the eggs, keep whisking.

- Pour the bowl of coconut oil, cream cheese, and eggs into the bowl of soy protein isolate, salt, and all their friends. Whisk everything until they combine and form together well.

- Pour in the apple cider vinegar. Stir it till it combines well.

- Add the chia and flax seed mixture. Stir them around to spread them out.

- Let the bowl's contents settle for 5 minutes. You are looking for it to thicken and not be too runny, but you also want most of the seeds to remain visible.

- Bake for 35 minutes.

Zero Carb Keto Bread

This recipe takes about 50 minutes to prepare and bake and makes 16 servings. It is very low fat but also has zero carbs. There are only 3 ingredients, so is a great recommendation for beginners.

- Calories: 38
- Carbs: 0 grams
- Fat: 2 grams
- Fiber: 0 grams
- Protein: 4 grams

What to Use

- 0.25 tsp of sea salt
- 0.50 cups of Soy protein isolate
- 6 large egg whites

Baking Instructions

- Preheat oven to 350F. While that is warming up get a baking pan and grease it up.
- Separate the egg white and yolks into two separate large bowls.
- Whip the egg whites for 5 minutes with an electric hand mixer.
- Now you can and the egg yolks into the bowl of whites.

- Add in the soy protein isolate and sea salt. Fold the mixture together but be gentle when doing to not deflate the egg whites or disturb the integrity of the structure.

- Transfer the contents into the baking pan.

- Bake for 45 minutes.

Keto Farmers Bread

This recipe takes about 110 minutes to prepare and bake and makes 20 servings.

- Calories: 33
- Carbs: 1 gram
- Fat: 2 grams
- Fiber: 4 grams
- Protein: 2 grams

What to Use

- 0.25 tsp of salt
- 2 Tbsp of apple cider vinegar
- 0.50 cups of water (boiling)
- 1.50 Tbsp of baking powder
- 6 tsp of psyllium husk powder
- 1 cup of potato oat fiber
- 4 medium eggs
- 2 cups of cream cheese

Baking Instructions

- Preheat oven to 302F. While that is warming up go and grab a baking pan.

- Grab a large bowl and place inside it the eggs and salt. Mix them together until they blend well.
- Add the cream cheese to the eggs and salt. Mix until they combine well.
- Grab another large bowl and place inside it the oat fiber, baking powder, and psyllium husk powder. Mix everything together until it blends well.
- Pour the contents from the bowl of oat fiber and his friends into the bowl of eggs. Mix everything together.
- Add the boiling water and vinegar. Pour the water slowly. Give it a minute to settle, then stir everything together.
- Let it settle and cool off for 15 minutes.
- When ready, use your hands to mold the dough into the shape of a bread loaf. Transfer the loaf onto the baking pan.
- Use some more of the oat fiber to place on top of the loaf (this will make the finished product look nice and white).
- Bake for 90 minutes.

Coconut Bread Loaf

This recipe takes about 45 minutes to prepare and bake and makes 8 servings.

- Calories: 135
- Carbs: 4 grams
- Fat: 9 grams
- Fiber: 64 grams
- Protein: 8 grams

What to Use

- 1 Tbsp of apple cinnamon vinegar
- 0.50 cup of water
- 0.50 tsp baking soda
- 1 tsp baking powder
- 1 tsp salt
- 0.50 cups of flaxseed meal
- 1 cup of coconut flour
- 6 large eggs

Baking Instructions

- Make sure oven is preheated to 350F. While that is warming up go and grab a loaf pan and grease it up.

- Place coconut flour in a mixing bowl and sift it, then place it in a large bowl.
- Add the baking soda, baking powder, salt, flaxseed meal. Whisk them together.
- Add the vinegar, water, and eggs.
- Stir the batter until it is nice and thick.
- Place the batter in baking pans. Bake it for 40 minutes.

Keto Coconut Flour Flatbread

This recipe takes about 15 minutes to prepare and bake and makes 6 servings.

- Calories: 66
- Carbs: 8 grams
- Fat: 3 grams
- Fiber: 5 grams
- Protein: 2 grams

What to Use

- 2 tsp of olive oil
- 0.25 tsp of salt
- 0.25 tsp of baking soda
- 1 cup of water (lukewarm)
- 0.50 cups of coconut flour
- 2 Tbsp of psyllium husk powder

Baking Instructions

- Grab a medium bowl and place inside it the coconut flour and psyllium husk powder
- Pour in the water, baking soda and only 1 tsp of the olive oil (the other half will be used later). Stir it all together until it mixes well.
- With your hands, knead the dough.

- Sprinkle the salt into the kneaded dough.

- Knead it again for 2 minutes.

- Let it settle for 10 minutes.

- When ready, separate the dough into 4 pieces. Roll each separate piece into a ball.

- Get two sheets of parchment paper and use a rolling pin to flatten the dough.

- Cut the bread into circular shapes. You will probably have extra dough from doing this. Use the extra dough to form 2 more balls.

- Flatten the 2 extra pieces of excess dough and cut them into circular shapes.

- Turn the stovetop on medium-high and get a skillet ready.

- Pour the rest of the olive oil into the skillet to oil up the pan.

- Place the flatbread dough into the pan (remove the parchment paper first).

- Cook for 3 minutes. Then flip the flatbread and cook the opposite sides for another 3 minutes.

Keto Sourdough Bread

This recipe takes about 90 minutes to prepare and bake and makes 12 servings.

- Calories: 369
- Carbs: 22 grams
- Fat: 30 grams
- Fiber: 16 grams
- Protein: 9 grams

What to Use

- 1 large egg white
- 5 large eggs
- 2 Tbsp of cream of tartar
- 1 Tbsp of salt
- 1 Tbsp of baking soda
- 0.25 cups of coconut flour
- 0.75 cups of almond flour
- 8 Tbsp of psyllium husk powder
- 0.50 cups of water (warm)
- 1.25 cups of almond nuts (blanched)

Baking Instructions

- Preheat the oven to 350F. While that is warming up go and grab a loaf pan and line it with parchment paper.
- Place the water and almond nuts in a blender. Blend for 2 minutes, until they smoothly come together. Pour it into a separate bowl and set it off to the side.
- Grab a large bowl and place inside it the salt, baking powder, psyllium husk powder, coconut flour, and almond flour. Mix everything till they combine well.
- Grab 2 more medium bowls and separate the egg yolks from all the egg whites. Fill both bowls with each (one bowl of yolk and another for the whites).
- Go get a small bowl. Take out one of the yolks and place it inside the small bowl. This will be used later for your egg wash.
- Place both bowls of egg yolk to the side for later use.
- Start beating the egg whites till they begin to soften. Add half of the cream of tartar to the mix, then continue beating for 1 more minute. Add the rest of the cream of tartar and beat again for another minute. Place the mixture off to the side for later use.
- Pour the egg yolks into the bowl of almond flour, coconut flour, and all their friends. Then transfer the entire mixture into an electric blender. Blend for 2 minutes or until everything comes together well.
- Pour the almond mixture into the blender and blend for another minute.

- Add the egg whites into the blender and blend slowly for 30 seconds.

- Transfer the contents into the baking pan. Return to the bowl with a single yolk and use that to brush the dough.

- Bake for 60 minutes.

Keto Lemon Blueberry Bread

This recipe takes about 200 minutes to prepare and bake and makes 10 servings.

The majority of the baking length is due to the cooldown time (2 hours). This is an approximate, maximum, time frame. You can check to see if the blueberries have cooled down after a half hour. By 2 hours, it should certainly have cooled off.

- Calories: 207
- Carbs: 21 grams
- Fat: 17 grams
- Fiber: 16 grams
- Protein: 9. grams

What to Use

- 1 cup of blueberries
- One large lemon (zested)
- 0.50 tsp of vanilla extract
- 1 Tbsp lemon extract
- 3 Tbsp of mayonnaise (dairy-free)
- 2 medium egg whites
- 6 large eggs
- 0.25 tsp of salt

- 0.50 tsp baking soda
- 1 tsp cream of tartar
- 0.25 cups of coconut flour
- 0.75 cups of stevia
- 2 cups of almond flour

Baking Instructions

- Preheat oven to 350F. While that is warming up go and get a bread pan and line it up with parchment paper.
- Get a large bowl and place inside the almond flour, coconut flour, baking soda, salt, and stevia. Whisk everything together till it combines.
- Add the eggs, egg whites, lemon zest, vanilla extract, lemon extract, and mayonnaise. Use an electric mixer to combine everything well.
- Add the blueberries to the mixture, but only use a third of them. Save the rest for later use. Stir until they mix in.
- Transfer the entire mixture of dough to the pan.
- Bake for 20 minutes.
- Take the dough out of the oven and top it with what is left of the blueberries.
- Bake for another 50 minutes.

- Remove from the oven and give it 2 hours to cool down. Yeah, that's the long part. You can check every thirty minutes to see if has cooled off. 2 hours is the maximum cooldown time.

Bulletproof Naan Keto Bread

This recipe takes about 30 minutes to prepare and bake and makes 8 servings.

- Calories: 30
- Carbs: 20 grams
- Fat: 22 grams
- Fiber: 4 grams
- Protein: 5 grams

What to Use

- 2 cloves of garlic (minced)
- 0.50 cups of butter
- 2 cups of water (boiling)
- 4 Tbsp of coconut oil
- 1 tsp of sea salt
- 0.50 tsp of baking powder
- 2 Tbsp of psyllium husk powder
- 0.75 cups of coconut flour

Baking Instructions

- Preheat the oven to 350F. While that is warming up go and grab a baking sheet and line it with parchment paper.

- Grab a large bowl and place inside it the coconut flour, psyllium husk powder, baking powder, and salt. Stir it all together.

- Add the coconut oil and then add the boiling water. Stir them thoroughly.

- Let the dough settle and rise for 5 minutes.

- Break the dough up into 8 separate pieces.

- Place the dough on the baking sheet and use a rolling pin or your hands to flatten them.

- Melt the butter in a microwave for 1 minute. When that's ready, add the minced garlic to the butter and stir it around. Give it 1 minute to gather together after stirring.

- Brush the dough with the butter and garlic. If desired, do not use all of the butter and garlic as a brush and save some to dip the Naan bread when you sit down to eat it.

- Bake for 20 minutes.

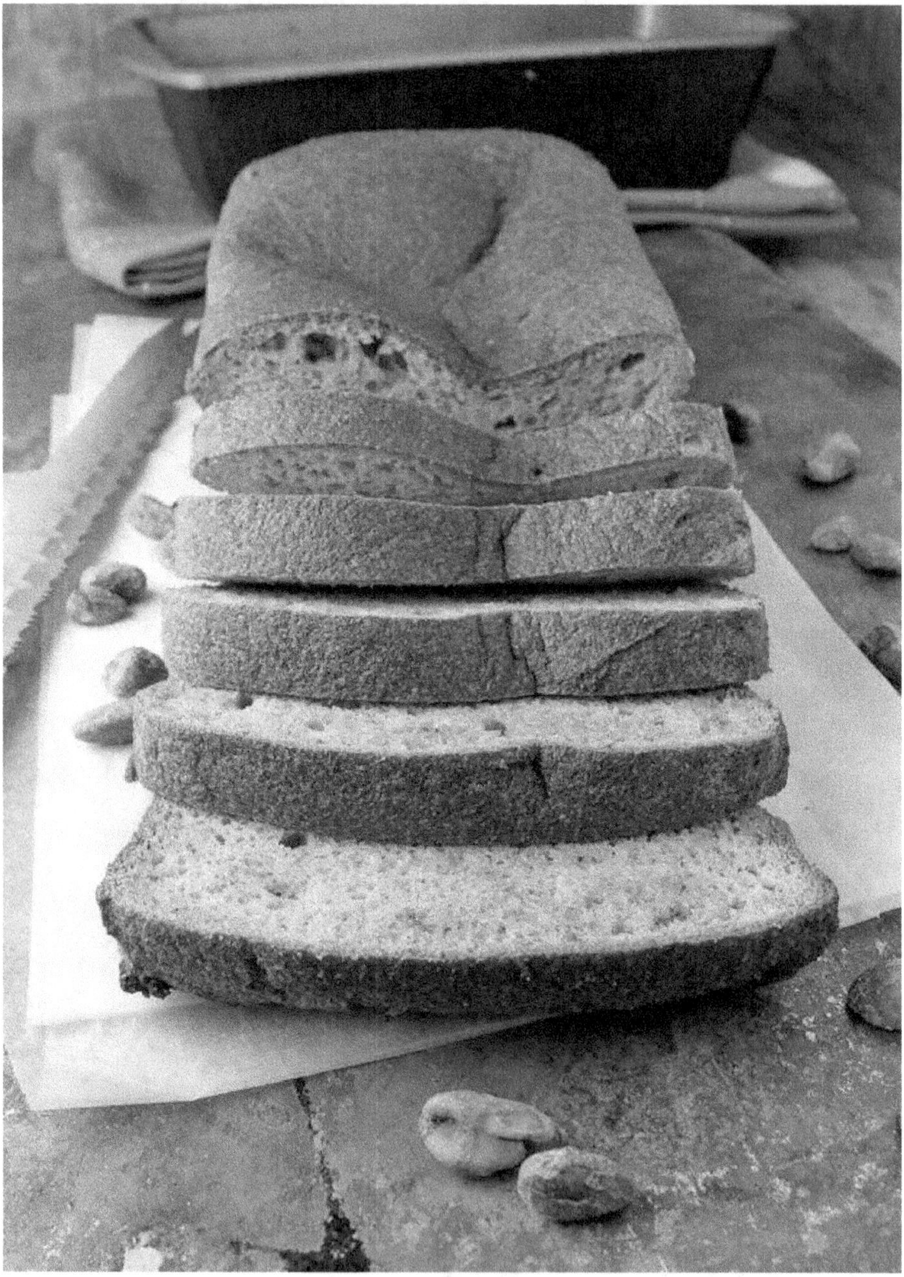

Pumpkin Bread Loaf

This recipe takes about 80 minutes to prepare and bake and makes 10 servings. This recipe contains stevia, but any non-sugar-based sweetener will work.

- Calories: 118
- Carbs: 6 grams
- Fat: 9 grams
- Fiber: 5 grams
- Protein: 5 grams

What do Use

- 0.50 tsp of sea salt
- 1.50 tsp of pumpkin pie spice
- 2 tsp baking powder
- 3 Tbsp of stevia
- 0.25 tsp of psyllium husk powder
- 0.50 cups coconut milk
- 0.50 cups pumpkin puree
- 3 large egg whites
- 1.50 cups almond flour
- 1 cup of water (warm)

Baking Instructions

- Preheat oven to 350F. Fill a baking dish with 1 cup of water. Place container with water on bottom rack. The water is used to generate steam to help the bread rise. Also, go get a loaf pan and grease it up.

- Place the psyllium husk powder, almond flour, swerve sweetener, baking powder, pumpkin spice, and salt into a large bowl. Mix everything together until it combines well.

- Add pumpkin puree and coconut milk into the same bowl and mix well.

- Whip egg whites in a second bowl.

- Fold about a third of the egg whites into the dough, mix it up. Then add the rest of the egg whites. When adding egg whites be careful and try not to deflate them.

- Transfer the dough into the pan.

- Bake for 75 minutes.

Walnut and Zucchini Loaf

This recipe takes about 70 minutes to prepare and bake and makes 16 servings.

- Calories: 200
- Carbs: 30 grams
- Fat: 20 grams
- Fiber: 3 grams
- Protein: 6 grams

What to Use

- 0.50 cups of walnuts (chopped)
- 1 cup of zucchini. Make sure that it is grated.
- 0.25 tsp of ground ginger
- 1 tsp of cinnamon (ground)
- 0.50 tsp of nutmeg
- 1.50 tsp of baking powder
- 0.50 tsp salt
- 1.50 cups of erythritol
- 2.50 cups of almond flour
- 1 tsp vanilla extract
- 8 Tbsp of olive oil

- 3 large eggs

Baking instructions

- Make sure oven is preheated to 350F. While that is warming up go and grab a loaf pan and grease it up.

- Put the vanilla extract, oils, and eggs into one large bowl. Whisk them together then put them to the side to use later.

- Place the ginger, nutmeg, salt, cinnamon, baking powder, almond flour, and erythritol into the second large bowl. Mix it all together and set aside.

- Get the (grated) zucchini ready by squeezing out any excess water it may have. A paper towel should be fine for this. Then add the zucchini to the bowl filled with eggs, vanilla, and oils. Whisk them all together.

- Pour the ingredients from the second bowl (the ginger, nutmeg, and all their friends) into the first bowl with the eggs and zucchini. Pour slowly and use a hand mixer to blend them all together.

- Using a spoon, transfer the mixture into the pan.

- Add the chopped walnuts and use a spoon or spatula to press them into the mixture.

- Bake for about 60 minutes. When the walnuts look browned, its ready to serve.

Flax Seed Bread

This recipe takes about 20 minutes to prepare and makes 8 servings.

This recipe contains stevia, but non-sugar-based sweetener would also do.

- Calories: 266
- Carbs: 6 grams
- Fat: 16 grams
- Fiber: 11 grams
- Protein: 24 grams

What to Use

- 1 cup of ground flax seed
- 1 large egg
- 7 large egg whites
- 4 Tbsp of Stevia
- 1.50 cups of soy protein isolate
- 1 Tbsp of baking powder
- 6 Tbsp of psyllium husk powder
- 3 Tbsp of butter

Baking Instructions

- Preheat oven to 350F. While that is warming up go and get a loaf pan and grease it up.

- Place the egg and butter, water, and egg whites into one large bowl. Mix them together and whisk.
- Place the salt, soy protein isolate, baking powder, and psyllium husk into a second large bowl.
- Pour the eggs, butter, and water into the bowl with the soy, baking powder, and other powders. Pour it slowly to mix everything together comfortably.
- Bake for about 20 minutes. This loaf is known to behave differently depending on the oven used. It may finish baking before twenty minutes, so keep an eye on it.

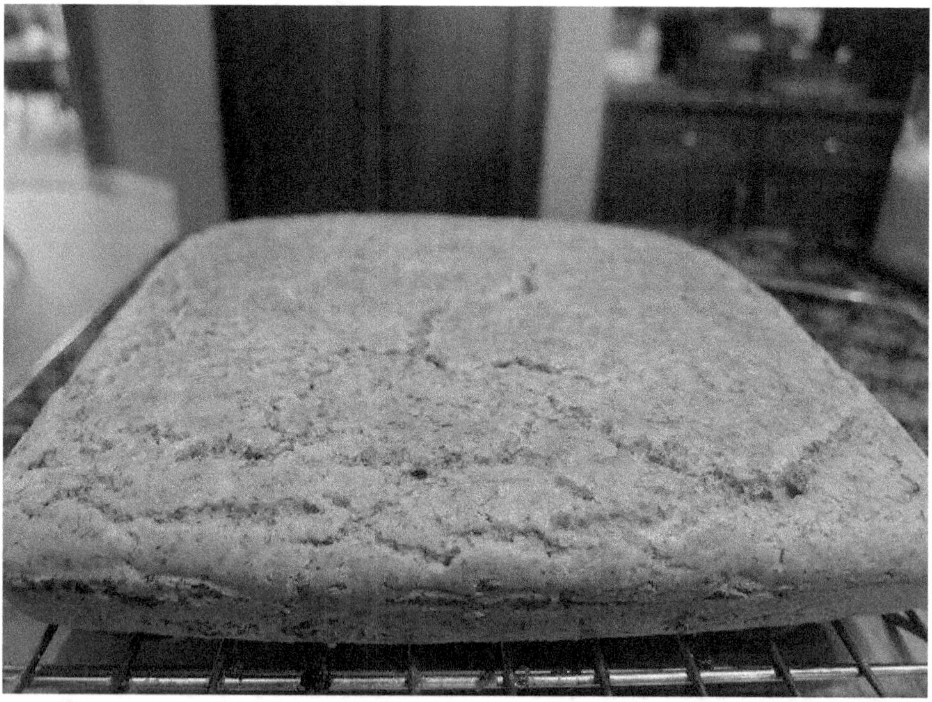

Keto Focaccia Bread

This recipe takes about 30 minutes to prepare and bake and makes 9 servings.

- Calories: 245
- Carbs: 4 grams
- Fat: 20 grams
- Fiber: 4 grams
- Protein: 10 grams

What to Use

- 1 tsp of red chili flakes
- 1 tsp of rosemary
- 1 tsp of salt
- 2 tsp of garlic. Make sure the garlic is finely minced.
- 1.50 Tbsp of baking powder
- 4 Tbsp of olive oil
- 1 cup of golden milled flaxseed
- 1 cup of almond flour
- 7 large eggs

Baking Instructions

- Preheat over to 350F. While that is warming up go and grab a baking pan and grease it up.

- In one medium bowl place the following; chili flakes, rosemary, salt, baking powder, flaxseed, almond flour. Mix them together thoroughly.

- Add the garlic. Mx it in.

- Add 2 eggs and mix them in. For the eggs, you may want to use a hand mixer for easier use. After mixing the 2 eggs in, add two more eggs and mix those. Then add two more eggs and mix those as well. Then add the final egg and mix that in. It Is recommended to add the eggs slowly to keep the dough stable for baking.

- Add in the olive oil and mix everything together a little more until it is nice and consistent, keeping the same stability and coloring throughout the batter.

- When done mixing place transfer the batter into the pan using a spoon.

- Bake for 25 minutes. Let cool for about 10 minutes.

Sesame Seed Keto Bread

This recipe takes about 65 minutes to prepare and bake and makes 6 servings.

- Calories: 100
- Carbs: 7 grams
- Fat: 13 grams
- Fiber: 6 grams
- Protein: 7 grams

What to Use

- 2 Tbsp of sesame seeds
- 5 Tbsp of psyllium husk powder
- 0.25 tsp of sea salt
- 2 tsp of apple cider vinegar
- 2 tsp baking powder
- 1.25 cups of almond flour
- 1 cup of boiling water
- 3 egg whites

Baking Instructions

- Preheat oven to 350F. Boil some water while you're at it. Also, go and grab a baking sheet and grease it up.

- Get a large bowl and toss in the sea salt, baking powder, almond flour, psyllium husk powder, and sesame seeds. Mix them all together.

- Add the water first (but make sure that it is boiling). Then add the apple cider vinegar and egg whites. Mix it well with a hand mixer, but for no longer than a minute. Overdoing the mixing may affect the integrity of the dough.

- Transfer the dough to the baking sheet.

- Bake for 60 minutes. Place the baking sheet on the lower rack when you do so. This is recommended for the seeds.

Rosemary and Lemon Low Carb Shortbread

This recipe takes about 50 minutes to prepare and bake and makes 24 servings.

Despite the name and appearance of this bread, it is still a healthy alternative when having guests over or looking for a wonderful snack. Stevia is in this recipe, but any non-sugar-based sweetener will do. This recipe can be a little tricky so read carefully.

- Calories: 80
- Carbs: 3 grams
- Fat: 7 grams
- Fiber: 1 gram
- Protein: 2 grams

What to Use

- 0.50 tsp of baking powder
- 0.50 tsp of baking soda
- 2 tsp of rosemary (fresh is the best)
- 1 tsp of vanilla extract
- 5 tsp of lemon juice (fresh squeezed is the best squeezed)
- 1 Tbsp of grated lemon zest (again, fresh is the best)
- 0.50 of Stevia
- 2 cups of almond flour

- 6 Tbsp of butter

Baking Instructions

- Get two separate bowls ready. One large, the other medium (and microwave safe). Also get some plastic wrap while you're at it.

- Take the almond flour, Stevia, baking soda, and baking powder and place it into the large bowl. Mix them together then set aside for later.

- Melt the butter (microwave is the fastest way) and add the vanilla extract to the melted butter. If using the microwave to melt the butter, then be sure to use a microwave-safe bowl.

- Take the contents from the large bowl and pour it into the medium one (this may seem counterintuitive but give it a try, and if it is not working then do the reverse and pour the contents from the medium bowl into the large).

- Now, with the large and empty bowl, add; lemon juice, lemon zest, butter with vanilla, and rosemary.

- Begin to stir and mix the lemon juice, zest, butter, and rosemary.

- While mixing, slowly pour the contents from the medium bowl (almond flour and his buddies) into the large bowl. Continue to mix while pouring slowly until all the contents of the medium bowl have entered the large one.

- When ready, wrap the dough in the plastic wrap you prepared earlier. Place the wrapped dough into the freezer. Let it solidify there for 30 minutes.

- After the thirty minutes has passed, preheat the oven to 350F. Retrieve the dough and unwrap it.

- Go get a sharp knife (that's what's best used to keep the structure of the dough intact). After thirty minutes in the freezer the dough should remain stable while being cut, but, if it does not then place it the freezer for a little longer. When confident the dough won't crumble, cut into sections about half an inch wide.

- Grease a cookie sheet with butter and put the sections you cut up on it. Bake for 15 minutes and let cool for 10.

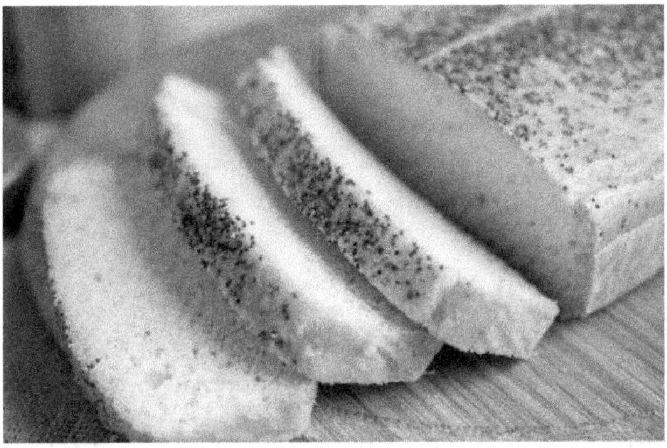

Keto Poppy Seed Almond Bread

This recipe takes about 75 minutes to prepare and bake and makes 14 servings.

- Calories: 227
- Carbs: 40 grams
- Fat: 12 grams
- Fiber: 2 grams
- Protein: 7 grams

What to Use

- 1 Tbsp of poppy seeds
- 0.50 cups of water
- 0.50 cups of avocado oil
- 0.50 tsp of pink Himalayan salt
- 2 tsp of baking powder
- 2 cups of blanched almond meal (ground)
- 5 large eggs

Baking Instructions

- Preheat oven to 400F. While the oven is warming up go grab a baking pan and place parchment paper on it.
- Place the salt, baking powder, and almond meal in a large bowl and mix them together.

- As you are mixing the salt, baking powder, and almond meal, you will also want to lightly drizzle the avocado oil into the mix. When the dough starts to take a powdery, crumbled like form, you will pierce a small hole through the center of the dough.

- Add the eggs to the mixture, then pour in the water. Stir the batter slowly with a hand mixer until it gives a light, yellowish, appearance.

- After the batter begins to take proper color and froth, stir faster to create bigger holes in the mix. Pour the almonds into the bigger holes that start to form from mixing. Continue to mix until the batter is smooth and thick.

- Pour the mix into a pan and casually drop the poppy seeds onto it.

- Bake it for 40 minutes and let cool for 30.

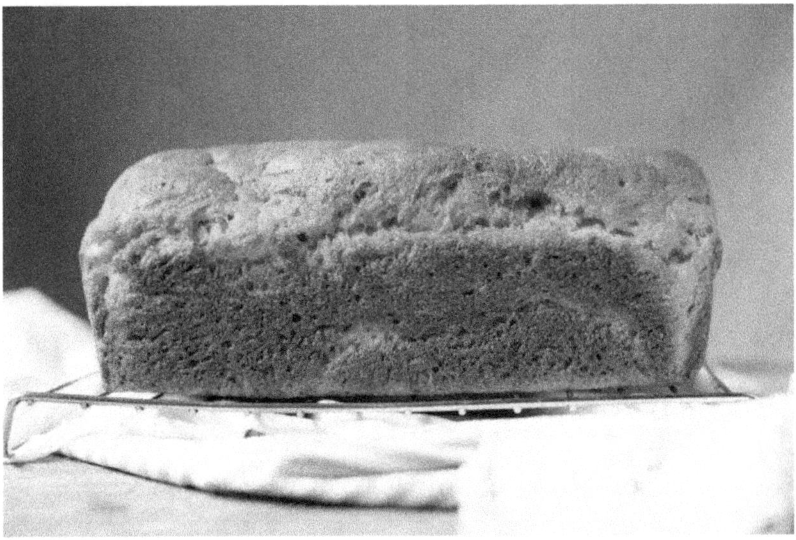

Keto Maple Bread

This recipe takes about 60 minutes to prepare and bake and makes 12 servings.

Don't let the word "maple" trick you into thinking this is non-keto. As the bread bakes the sugar will be cooked out of the finished product.

- Calories: 174
- Carbs: 6 grams
- Fat: 14 grams
- Fiber: 4 grams
- Protein: 5 grams

What to Use

- 0.25 cup of sour cream
- 1 Tbsp apple cinnamon vinegar
- 0.25 cups of butter
- 1 egg
- 3 egg whites
- 0.25 tsp of ground ginger
- 0.25 tsp of cream of tartar
- 1 tsp of sea salt
- 2 tsp of baking powder

- 2 tsp of xanthan gum
- 2 tsp of psyllium husks
- 0.25 cups of soy protein isolate
- 0.75 cups of golden flaxseed meal
- 0.25 cups of arrowroot flour
- 0.50 cups of water (warm)
- 2 tsp of active dry yeast
- 2 tsp of maple syrup

Baking Instructions

- First, heat up some water to about 105F. Then go grab a pan and line it up with parchment paper. Set it aside, you'll need it later.
- Heat up some butter to melt it in the microwave, then let it cool down.
- Place the maple syrup and yeast into a large bowl.
- Pour water over the yeast and syrup mixture, then cover it. A regular kitchen towel should do. Let it rest for 8 minutes.
- While the magic of yeast proofing is happening, go get a medium bowl. Mix into it the ginger, cream of tartar, flaxseed meal, arrowroot flour, salt, baking powder, xanthan gum, whey protein powder and psyllium husk. Set that aside and return your attention to the yeast as it should be done proofing.

- The yeast should be done proofing. So, it's time to add the egg, egg whites, butter, and vinegar. Use an electric mixer for about two minutes until it froths and is light in appearance.

- Add only half of the contents from the medium bowl, then toss in the sour cream, mixing as you do so. Then add the other half of the contents from the medium bowl. Mix it up quickly and be thorough to make sure the xanthan gum is activated.

- Place the dough into the pan you prepared earlier with parchment paper. The top may be uneven, and if so, the smooth it out with a spatula.

- Give it some time for the dough to naturally rise, about 50 minutes. Preheat the oven to 350 while waiting. Since the dough for this recipe is rising naturally, keep an eye on it to make sure it does not rise past the height of the pan.

- Place a baking tray in the oven and put the pan of the loaf on top of it.

- Bake for 55 minutes. Around the 15-minute mark, you may want to cover it loosely with a dome of foil. This is to prevent the rising from getting out of hand.

- Let cool for five minutes.

Keto Stuffed Savory Bread

This recipe takes about 55 minutes to prepare and bake and makes 12 servings.

- Calories: 202
- Carbs: 5 grams
- Fat: 20 grams
- Fiber: 3 grams
- Protein: 6 grams

What to Use

- 1.50 tsp of baking powder
- 2 Tbsp of parsley seasoning
- 1 tsp of sage seasoning
- 1 tsp of rosemary seasoning
- 8 medium eggs
- 1 cup of cream cheese
- 0.50 cups of butter
- 0.25 cups of coconut flour
- 2.5 cups of almond flour

Baking Instructions

- Preheat oven to 350F. While that is warming up go and grab a loaf pan. Grease up the loaf pan.

- Grab a medium bowl and place inside it the cream cheese and butter. Stir them together until they combine well.

- Add the seasoning of rosemary, sage, and parsley. Whip them together until they combine well.

- Place the eggs inside the batter and continue to whip everything together until a batter takes form. The appearance should look smooth.

- Add the baking powder, coconut flour, and almond flour. Stir it together until the batter appears thick.

- Bake for 50 minutes.

Low Carb Keto Banana Bread

This recipe takes about 80 minutes to prepare and bake and makes 16 servings.

Now, bananas may not be known as the best food to use on a low carb or keto diet, but if you wanted to give it a try, have a special event, or just love banana bread, here it is. Despite all that, this recipe is designed to be low in carbs anyway. This recipe also contains stevia, but any non-sugar-based sweetener will work.

- Calories: 165
- Carbs: 10 grams
- Fat: 15 grams
- Fiber: 2 grams
- Protein: 4 grams

What to Use

- 1 tsp of baking powder
- 0.25 tsp of stevia.
- 0.50 tsp of salt
- 0.50 tsp of xanthan gum
- 0.33 cups of coconut flour
- 0.75 cups of almond flour
- 1 tsp of vanilla extract
- 6 medium eggs

- 0.50 cups of erythritol
- 3 Tbsp of coconut oil
- 0.50 cups of butter (melted)
- 1 medium banana (smashed all up and mushy)

Baking Instructions

- Preheat oven to 325F. While that is warming up grab a loaf pan and grease it up.
- Go get a medium bowl and place inside it the baking powder, erythritol, stevia, salt, xanthan gum, coconut flour, and almond flour. Mix them all up until they combine well. Set the bowl aside for later.
- Grab a food processor and place inside it the vanilla extract, eggs, coconut oil, butter, and mashed up banana. Pulse for about 1 minute until everything blends together nicely.
- Add the contents from the bowl of the flours and all their friends into the food processor. Pulse for another minute until the batter blends together well.
- Transfer the batter from the food processor into the loaf pan.
- Bake for 75 minutes.

Chapter 5: Bagel Time

Oh, bagels, what would our mornings (or lunches or dinners) be without you? Bagels are another one of the foods that many people fear giving up when trying to go Keto, but with these recipes, you won't have to worry about giving up one of the most popular staples of food the world over.

Poppy and Sesame Seed Bagels

This recipe takes about 25 minutes to prepare and bake and makes 6 servings.

- Calories: 350
- Carbs: 8 grams
- Fat: 29 grams
- Fiber: 3 grams
- Protein: 20 grams

What to Use

- 8 tsp of sesame cheese
- 8 tsp of poppy seeds
- 0.25 cups of cream cheese
- 2.50 cups of shredded mozzarella cheese
- 1 tsp of baking powder

- 1. 5 cups of almond flour
- 2 large eggs

Baking Instructions

- Preheat oven to 400F. While that is warming up go and grab a baking sheet and place parchment paper on top of it.
- In a medium bowl combine the baking powder and almond flour. Mix them together till they blend.
- Melt the cream cheese and mozzarella together in a separate medium (and microwave safe) bowl. 2 minutes should do the trick. However, stop after only 1 minute and make sure that you stir the cheese. Then heat it for another minute.
- Beat the eggs. Then add the eggs to the bowl of cream cheese and mozzarella.
- Combine the contents from both bowls together. Mix them all together until the dough begins to mix well.
- Break or cut the dough up into 6 separate pieces.
- Stretch the dough and interlock the 2 opposite ends to give the dough a proper bagel shape.
- Place the bagels onto the baking sheet.
- Take the poppy and sesame seeds and press them into the bagel dough.
- Bake for 15 minutes.

Fathead Dough Bagels

This recipe takes about 27 minutes to prepare and bake and makes 6 servings.

This may seem similar to the previous recipe but the major difference, aside from lack of seeds, is that the dough is fathead dough. For fathead dough you will need to mold and knead the dough with your hands, so make sure they are nice and clean, and also make sure you are ready to get a bit messy. This is something to keep in mind when making fathead dough. Fathead is not the only dough that you use your hands with, but it is one of its traits. Fathead dough can be very sticky as well, and some people find it difficult to work with.

- Calories: 360
- Carbs: 8 grams
- Fat: 28 grams
- Fiber: 3 grams
- Protein: 21 grams

What to Use

- 2 large eggs
- 3 Tbsp of cream cheese
- 2.50 cups of mozzarella cheese
- 1 Tbsp of baking powder
- 1.50 cups of almond flour

Baking Instructions

- Preheat oven to 400F. While it is warming up go and get a baking pan and line it up with some parchment paper.

- Place the almond flour and baking powder in a medium bowl and stir them up together. Set it aside for now.

- Melt the cream cheese and mozzarella together in a separate medium (and microwave safe) bowl. 2 minutes should do the trick. However, stop after only 1 minute and make sure that you stir the cheese. Then heat it for another minute.

- For the following step, you will have to work with haste as you want to get everything going while the cheese is still hot.

- Put the eggs and almond flour/baking soda into the melted cheese. Then knead with your hands until the dough starts to take proper form. It will be sticky so make sure you continue to work through it and knead the dough before it starts to harden.

- If by chance it does, unfortunately, begin to harden before you have finished kneading it, then place it back in the microwave. Only heat it for 15-20 seconds. Then knead again, but make sure you have washed your hands first (remember that warning above about things getting messy. Consider it a light form of collateral damage that goes with cooking and baking).

- Take note, when kneading the dough of this type, you must make extra sure that everything is smooth and uniform throughout. This may seem obvious, but it is worth taking an extra look to make sure that everything comes out properly. Try to notice if any of the cheese and almond flour is separated, as it shouldn't be. If it needs more kneading, then make sure you do that and bring everything together properly. After examining the dough and making sure that everything in uniform, you may continue.

- Break the dough up into 6 separate sections and roll the individual sections into long log shapes, then interlock the two opposing ends to create a proper bagel shape. If it is too difficult, then place it on the baking sheet and roll the dough into the shapes of bagels there.

- Place the bagels on the baking sheet.

- Bake for 15 minutes.

Keto Everything Bagel

This recipe takes about 30 minutes to prepare and bake and makes 6 servings.

- Calories: 449
- Carbs: 10 grams
- Fat: 36 grams
- Fiber:4 grams
- Protein: 27 grams

What to Use

- 3 Tbsp of Everything seasoning
- 5 Tbsp of cream cheese
- 3 cups of mozzarella cheese (shredded)
- 3 large eggs
- 1 tsp of Italian seasoning (dried)
- 1 tsp of onion powder
- 1 tsp of garlic powder
- 1 Tbsp of baking powder
- 2 cups of almond flour

Baking Instructions

- Preheat oven to 425F. While that is warming up go and get a baking sheet and line it with parchment paper.

- Go grab a medium mixing bowl. Place inside the Italian seasoning, onion powder, garlic powder, baking powder, and almond flour. Mix them all up together.

- In a small bowl, crack and place only one of the eggs. Whisk it up. This egg will not go into the dough but will be used for egg wash to brush the top of the bagels.

- Melt the cream cheese and mozzarella together in a separate medium (and microwave safe) bowl. 2 minutes should do the trick. However, stop after only 1 minute and make sure that you stir the cheese. Then heat it for another minute.

- Give your attention back to the medium mixing bowl with the powders, Italian seasoning, and almond flour. Add the reaming 2 eggs to the mix and stir it up nice and good. If the dough becomes tough, heat it in the microwave for 30 seconds and continue to mix it up.

- Break the dough up into 6 separate pieces and roll the portions int a ball.

- Stretch the dough out into long log-like shapes. Interlock the two opposing ends to create the proper bagel shape.

- Gently brush up the tops of the bagels with the wash from the first egg you cracked, whisked, and set aside.

- Use the Everything seasoning to sprinkle atop each bagel individually.
- Bake for 14 minutes.

Cheesy Keto Bagels

This recipe takes about 32 minutes to prepare and bake and makes 6 servings.

- Calories: 35
- Carbs: 10 grams
- Fat: 65 grams
- Fiber: 25 grams
- Protein: 23 grams

What to Use

- 2 tsp of sesame seeds
- 4 Tbsp of cream cheese
- 2.5 cups of mozzarella (shredded)
- 3 large eggs
- 1 tsp of baking soda
- 2 tsp of cream of tartar
- 1 cup of coconut flour
- 1.5 cups of almond flour

Baking Instructions

- Preheat over to 400F. While that is warming up go and grab a pan to bake with and line it up with parchment paper.

- Grab a large bowl and place inside it the baking soda, cream of tartar, coconut flour, and almond flour. Whisk them all together.

- Melt the cream cheese and mozzarella together in a separate medium (microwave safe) bowl. 2 minutes should do the trick. However, stop after only 1 minute and make sure that you stir the cheese. Then heat it for another minute.

- Then grab a separate large bowl and break two eggs, toss them inside and whisk them up.

- Add those two whisked eggs to the bowl of flours, baking soda, and cream of tartar. Whisk them all up together.

- Add the cheese to the bowl that you just used. Make sure your hands are nice and clean, then use them to knead the dough together. Continue to do so until everything combines well.

- Divide the dough into 6 separate portions.

- Roll the 6 sections into the shape of long logs. Interlock the two opposing ends of the dough for each piece, so it creates the proper bagel shape.

- In a separate bowl break and whisk the final egg to make the egg wash. Brush the top of the bagels with it.

- Bake for 17 minutes.

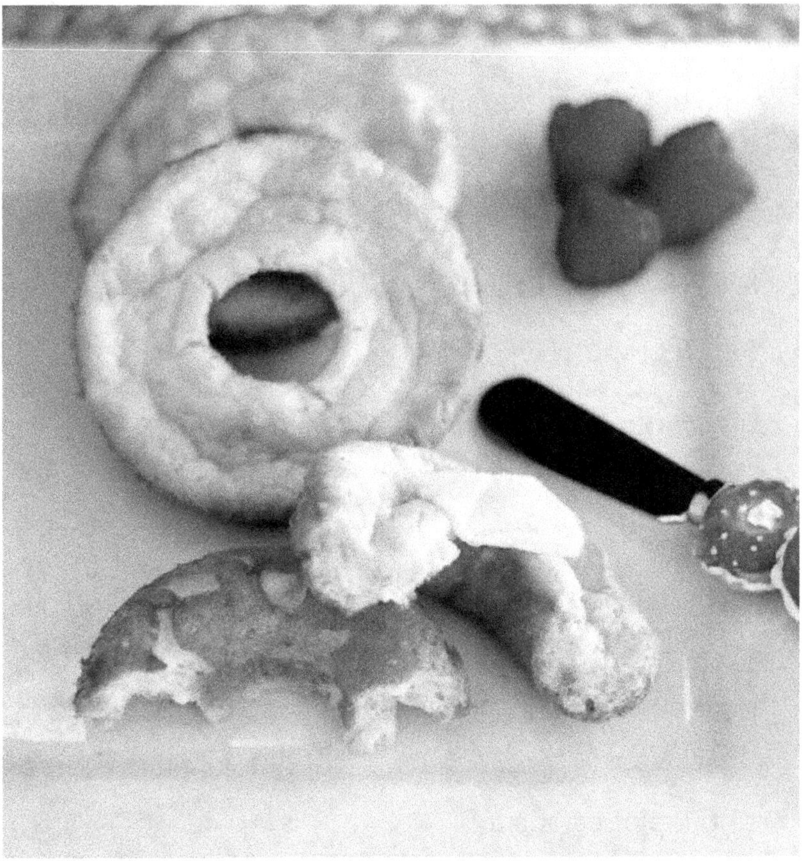

Low Carb Croissant Bagel

This recipe takes about 25 minutes to prepare and bake and makes 7 servings.

- Calories: 83
- Carbs: 3 grams
- Fat: 6 grams
- Fiber: 0.7 grams
- Protein: 3 grams

What to Use

- 0.125 tsp of sea salt
- 0.50 tsp of baking soda and 0.25 tsp of cream of tartar (mix them together beforehand)
- 1.50 tsp of erythritol
- 2 Tbsp of coconut flour
- 2 Tbsp of butter (make sure it is melted)
- 2 Tbsp of cream cheese
- 0.25 tsp of cream of tartar
- 3 medium eggs

Baking Instructions

- Preheat oven to 300F. Go grab a pan to bake with and grease it up. Also, be sure to melt the butter.

- Break the eggs and make sure to separate the yolk from the whites. Then place them in different bowls, one for the yolk and another for the whites. You can use a large bowl for each.

- Add the egg whites and cream of tartar together. Use a mixer to whip them together. The appearance should be stiff looking. Set it aside for later use.

- For the yolks, beat them and then combine the cream cheese, sea salt, erythritol, cream of tartar, baking soda, coconut flour, and melted butter. Beat them together until they start to take form together.

- Fold the mixture of egg yolk into the mixture of egg whites. Be careful to be gentle when doing so. Try not to stir it around but combine them well.

- Use a spoon to transfer the mixture onto the baking sheet. Spread it around and make a hole for the regular bagel appearance.

- Bake for 20 minutes.

Garlic Coconut Flour Bagels

This recipe takes about 20 minutes to prepare and bake and makes 6 servings.

- Calories: 90
- Carbs: 6 grams
- Fat: 16 grams
- Fiber: 3 grams
- Protein: 8 grams

What to Use

- 0.5 tsp of baking powder
- 0.5 tsp of salt
- 1.5 tsp of garlic powder
- 2 tsp of xanthan gum
- 0.50 cups of coconut flour
- 0.75 cups of butter
- 6 medium eggs

Baking Instructions

- Preheat oven to 400F. Grease up a pan while it is heating up.
- Grab a large bowl and place the garlic powder, salt, butter, and eggs inside. Blend them all together.

- In a separate large bowl mix together the xanthan gum, baking powder, and coconut flour.
- Combine the contents from both bowls together by whisking the baking powder mixture into the egg bowl. There should be no lumps left after whisking.
- Use a spoon to transfer the batter into the pan.
- Bake for 15 minutes and let cool for 5.

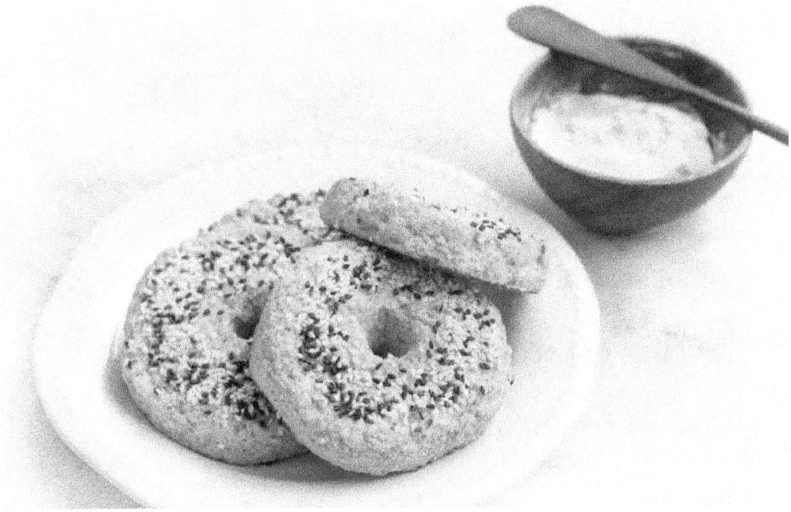

Keto Cauliflower Low Carb Bagels

This recipe takes about 38 minutes to prepare and bake and makes 4 servings.

- Calories: 107
- Carbs: 11 grams
- Fat: 4 grams
- Fiber: 6 grams
- Protein: 7 grams

What to Use

- 1 tsp of garlic powder
- 1 tsp of sea salt
- 0.25 cups of coconut flour
- 3 Tbsp of ground flaxseed
- 3 egg whites
- 1 single bag of riced cauliflower (frozen).

Baking Instructions

- Preheat oven to 375F. Grease a baking sheet while the oven is warming up.
- Either heat up the cauliflower in a microwave for 5 minutes or steam it in a pot for 8 minutes using medium heat.

- After the cauliflower is done cooking, add the coconut flour and ground flax. Stir it all up nice and well.

- Then add the garlic powder, salt, and egg whites. Stir it all up until the eggs are incorporated nicely.

- Break up the mixture into 8 separate pieces.

- Stretch the bagels out and interlock the two opposing ends to create the proper bagel shape.

- Place the bagels onto the baking sheet you greased earlier.

- Bake for 25 minutes.

- Take out of the oven, flip the bagels over for 5 minutes, then send them back in the oven for another 5 minutes.

Keto French Toast Bagel

This recipe takes about 25 minutes to prepare and bake and makes 6 servings.

Stevia is in this recipe, but any non-sugar-based sweetener will work.

- Calories: 207
- Carbs: 7 grams
- Fat: 16 grams
- Fiber: 4 grams
- Protein: 8 grams

What to Use

- 0.50 tsp of baking powder
- 0.50 tsp of xanthan gum
- 0.50 cups of coconut flour
- 0.50 tsp of salt
- 1 tsp of Stevia
- 1 tsp of maple extract
- 2 tsp of vanilla extract
- 1 Tbsp of cinnamon
- 6 medium eggs
- 3 Tbsp of butter (melted)

Baking Instructions

- Preheat oven at 400F. While that is warming up grab a pan and grease it up. Also, make sure to melt the butter while you're at it.

- Grab a large bowl and toss in the butter, eggs, salt, stevia, maple extract, vanilla extract, and cinnamon.

- In a separate medium bowl mix together the xanthan gum, baking powder, and coconut flour.

- Combine the mixture of coconut flour and egg batter. Whisk them together until there are no lumps left.

- Stretch the bagel dough into long logs and then interlock the two opposing ends to create the proper bagel shape.

- Transfer the bagel dough onto the greased baking pan.

- Bake for 15 minutes.

Keto Blueberry Cheesecake Bagels

This recipe takes about 25 minutes to prepare and bake and makes 11 servings.

- Calories: 196
- Carbs: 10 grams
- Fat: 13 grams
- Fiber: 1 gram
- Protein: 10 grams

What to Use

- 2 tsp of erythritol (this will be used in two separate places, so separate it)
- 1 Tbsp of baking powder
- 0.50 cups of blueberries
- 3 medium eggs
- 4 Tbsp of cream cheese
- 12 Tbsp of nut flour
- 0.75 cups of almond flour
- 2.50 cups of mozzarella cheese (shredded)

Baking Instructions

- Preheat oven to 400F.

- Melt the cream cheese and mozzarella together in a separate large (and microwave safe) bowl. 2 minutes should do the trick. However, stop after only 1 minute and make sure that you stir the cheese. Then heat it for another minute.

- Grab a second large bowl and mix in 1 tsp of the erythritol, baking powder, almond flour, and nut flour.

- Add 2 eggs to the bowl of melted cheese. Mix it up nice and well.

- Take the flour mixture and carefully pour it into the cheese and eggs combination.

- Knead the mixture together. Keep doing so until everything combines well.

- Fold in the blueberries. Do so carefully.

- Break the dough up into 8 sections.

- Stretch the bagel dough into long logs and then interlock the two opposing ends to create the proper bagel shape.

- Use the egg wash to brush the bagels.

- Bake for 15 minutes.

Low Carb Keto Onion Bagels

This recipe takes about 45 minutes to prepare and bake and makes 6 servings.

- Calories: 78
- Carbs: 3 grams
- Fat: 5 grams
- Fiber: 2 grams
- Protein: 5 grams

What to Use

- 1 tsp of onion's mined (and dried)
- 0.50 tsp of baking powder
- 0.125 cups of coconut flour
- 0.1875 cups of flaxseed meal
- 4 medium eggs

Baking Instructions

- Preheat oven to 325F. Get out a baking pan and spray or grease it up. Also, separate the egg whites from egg yolk.
- Grab a small bowl and put in the onion, baking powder, coconut flour, and flax meal. Mix it up nice and well.

- An electric mixer would be best for this next step of beating the egg whites until they give off a light and foamy appearance.
- Whisk the yolks.
- Add the yolks to the mixture of flax seed, coconut flour, baking soda, and onions. Set the batter off to the side and give it about 3 minutes to settle itself.
- Transfer the dough onto the pan. If you would like, add some more dried onion on top.
- Bake for 30 minutes.

Low Carb Keto Pumpkin Bagel

This recipe takes about 33 minutes to prepare and bake and makes 8 servings.

- Calories: 82
- Carbs: 5 grams
- Fat: 5 grams
- Fiber: 3 grams
- Protein: 3 grams

What to Use

- 1.5 Tbsp of erythritol
- 0.125 tsp of sea salt
- 0.50 tsp of cinnamon
- 1.25 pumpkin pie spice
- 1 tsp of vanilla extract
- 0.50 tsp of baking soda
- 1 tsp of apple cider vinegar
- 0.50 cups of pumpkin puree
- 0.25 cups of unsweetened coconut milk
- 2 Tbsp of melted coconut oil
- 3 medium eggs

- 3 Tbsp of golden flaxseed
- 0.75 cups of coconut flour

Baking Instructions

- Preheat oven to 350F. While it's warming up get a pan and grease it up.
- Get a large mixing bowl and place inside it the sea salt, cinnamon, pumpkin pie spice, golden flaxseed meal, and coconut flour. Mix it all together and set aside.
- Get a second large bowl and place inside it the coconut oil, erythritol, vanilla extract, coconut milk, pumpkin puree, and eggs. Mix them all together.
- Grab a pinch bowl and combine the baking soda and apple cider vinegar together.
- Add the apple cider vinegar, and baking soda to the egg mixture then stir them together.
- Add the egg mix to the bowl with coconut flour and then stir the batter. Continue to stir until the batter is smooth.
- Stretch the bagel dough into long logs and then interlock the two opposing ends to create the proper bagel shape.
- Transfer the bagel batter onto the pan.
- Bake for 25 minutes.

Keto Mozzarella Dough Bagels

This recipe takes about 25 minutes to prepare and bake and makes 6 servings.

- Calories: 203
- Carbs: 4 grams
- Fat: 17 grams
- Fiber: 12 grams
- Protein: 11 grams

What to Use

- 0.25 tsp of sea salt
- 1 tsp of baking powder
- 1 medium egg
- 2 Tbsp of cream cheese
- 0.75 cups of almond flour
- 1.75 cups of mozzarella cheese (shredded)

Baking Instructions

- Preheat oven to 425F. While that is warming up go and grab a baking tray.
- Go grab a large bowl (microwave safe) and place inside it the almond flour, cream cheese, and mozzarella. Heat them up in the microwave for 1 minute.

- Remove the bowl and stir the ingredients till they combine well. Then microwave for another 30 seconds.
- Add the salt, baking soda, and egg to the bowl.
- Separate the dough into 6 pieces.
- Stretch the bagel dough into long logs and then interlock the two opposing ends to create the proper bagel shape.
- Bake for 15 minutes.

Chapter 6: Keto Buns

Who doesn't want a nice and tasty bun now and then? Burgers, breakfast sandwiches, hot dogs, all classics that do not have to be sacrificed just because you are going on a keto diet. Yes, you could always have a burger without a bun, but isn't it nice knowing that you don't have to anymore and that there are options available? Combine these recipes with some grass-fed premium (or wild caught) meat and leave the guilt behind.

Keto Low Carb Hamburger Buns

This recipe takes about 23 minutes to prepare and bake and makes 5 servings.

- Calories: 294
- Carbs: 7 grams
- Net Carbs: 4 grams
- Fat: 25 grams
- Fiber: 3 grams
- Protein: 14 grams

What to Use

- 1 Tbsp of baking powder
- 1.50 cups of almond flour
- 4 Tbsp of cream cheese
- 1.5 cups of skim mozzarella cheese (grated)
- 1 large egg

Baking Instructions

- Preheat oven to 400F. While that is heating up grab a food processor (a blender is not recommended for this recipe unless it has the "pulse" setting). Also get a baking sheet and line it with parchment paper.
- Place both the cream cheese and mozzarella in a large (microwave safe) bowl and heat it up for 1 minute. Stir it up and then microwave it for another

30 seconds (keep in mind that microwaves vary so adjust accordingly). Transfer the melted cheese into a food processor, then process it until it has a smooth appearance.

- Take the egg, almond flour, baking powder, and toss all of them inside the processor. Process all of it along with the cheese until it forms into a dough. The dough should be sticky and may need to cool for 3 minutes.

- When the dough is ready, use your hands to break it up into 5 pieces.

- Roll the broken sections into ball shapes and place them on the baking pan. Depending on how the balls of dough look, you may want to flatten them out after placing them on the baking sheet but be careful not to make them too flat. They should retain a dome-like shape.

- To help the dough rise correctly, an extra trick is recommended here. Place a metal pan at the bottom of the oven and put 5 ice cubes inside. Place the baking sheet with the dough in the oven above it.

- Bake for 12 minutes.

Ultimate Keto Buns

This recipe takes about 60 minutes to prepare and bake and makes 10 servings.

- Calories: 208
- Carbs: 13 grams
- Fat: 15 grams
- Fiber: 8 grams
- Protein: 10 grams

What to Use

- 2 cups of water (warm)
- 6 large egg whites
- 2 tsp of apple cider vinegar
- 1 tsp of erythritol
- 5 Tbsp of sesame seeds
- 1 tsp of sea salt
- 1 tsp of baking soda
- 2 tsp of onion powder
- 2 tsp of garlic powder
- 0.3125 cups of flaxseed meal
- 0.50 cups of coconut flour

- 8 Tbsp of psyllium husk powder
- 1.5 cups of almond flour

Baking Instructions

- Preheat oven to 350F. While that is heating up go get a baking tray and line it with parchment paper.
- Go grab a large bowl and place inside it the erythritol, salt, baking soda, onion powder, garlic powder, flaxseed meal, coconut flour, and almond flour. Mx them all together until they blend well.
- In a separate bowl place inside it the psyllium husk powder, water, apple cider vinegar, and egg whites.
- Pour the contents (egg whites, water, husk powder, vinegar) from the second bowl into the first bowl.
- Mix everything up until well-combined. An electric hand mixer is recommended for this. The dough should have a thick appearance.
- Spoon out the buns and place them on the baking tray. Spread and press the sesame seeds onto and into the buns.
- Bake for 50 minutes. Let cool for 5.

Keto Seed-Splosion Buns

This recipe takes about 40 minutes to prepare and bake and makes 5 servings.

- Calories: 236
- Carbs: 8 grams
- Fat: 201 grams
- Fiber: 5 grams
- Protein: 8 grams

What to Use

- 3 Tbsp of Coconut oil (melted)
- 1 Tbsp of apple cider vinegar
- 2 medium egg whites
- 1 medium egg
- 0.50 tsp of garlic powder
- 0.50 tsp of Himalayan salt
- 1 tsp of black chia seeds
- 2 tsp of sunflower seeds
- 1 tsp of white sesame seeds
- 1 tsp of black sesame seeds
- 1 tsp of baking powder

- 2 Tbsp of psyllium husk powder
- 0.50 cups of blanched almond flour
- 4 Tbsp of water (boiling)

Baking Instructions

- Preheat oven to 350F. Grab a baking tray and line it with parchment paper.
- Place the almond flour, psyllium husk powder, baking powder, black sesame seeds, white sesame seeds, sunflower seeds, chia seeds, salt, and garlic powder in a large bowl. Whisk it all up until it combines well.
- In a separate large bowl place, the egg yolk, egg whites, apple cider vinegar, and melted coconut oil. Mix them up until they form together.
- Pour the contents from the second bowl (eggs and all their friends) into the first bowl with all the seeds, flour, and powders. Mix them all together until they combine well.
- Pour the water, boiling, into the mix. Since it's boiling, be sure to pour it slowly and carefully. After the water is in there, continue mixing it all up. The dough should give off a thick appearance.
- The batter may be sticky so give it a few minutes to settle if need be. When ready, use your hands to separate the dough into 5 pieces and roll them into balls. Then place the balls of dough onto the parchment paper and baking tray.
- Bake for 30 minutes.

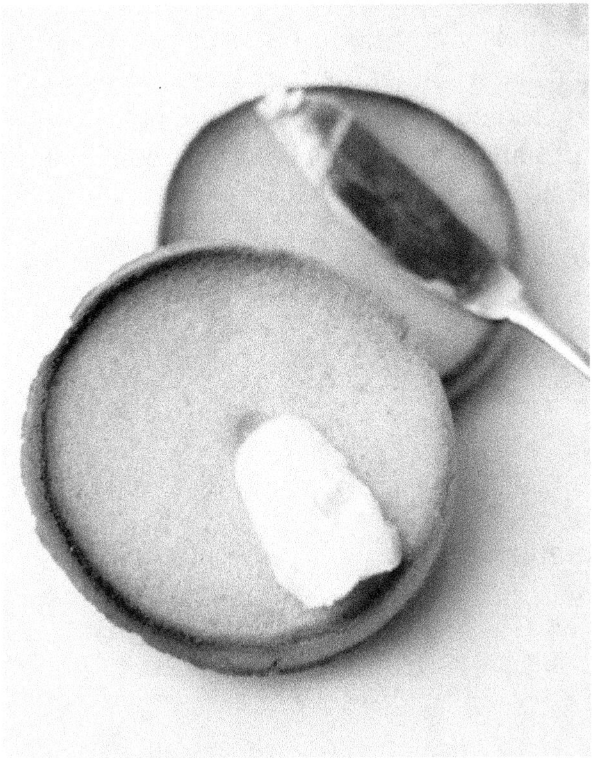

Muffin Keto Bun

This recipe takes about 32 minutes to prepare and bake and makes 6 servings. The name may have the word "muffin" but don't be fooled by that. This recipe is a bit different as the only appliance you will need are silicone muffin molds and immersion blender.

- Calories: 76
- Carbs: 4 grams
- Fat: 21 grams
- Fiber: 2 grams
- Protein: 9 grams

What to Use

- 1 tsp of onion flakes
- 1 Tbsp of white sesame seeds
- 1 Tbsp of black sesame seeds
- 1 Tbsp of rosemary
- 1.50 cups of almond flour (blanched)
- 0.50 tsp of pink Himalayan salt
- 4 medium eggs
- 4 Tbsp of butter (melted)

Baking Instructions

- Preheat oven to 430F.

- Place the eggs and melted butter inside the immersion blender. Pulse them 2 or 3 times.
- Then add the salt, almond flour, rosemary, both types of sesame seeds, and onion flakes.
- Pulse everything in the immersion blender 6 to 10 times. All the batter should be mixed together nicely.
- Take the muffin molds (silicone, metal is not recommended for this recipe) and pour the batter into 6 places.
- Bake for 26 minutes.

Keto Almond Buns

This recipe takes about 20 minutes to prepare and bake and makes 3 servings.

This is another recipe that does not contain many ingredients and is quick to the point, so it's great for beginners. It does contain stevia, but any non-sugar-based sweetener will work.

- Calories: 373
- Carbs: 7 grams
- Fat: 35 grams
- Fiber: 3 grams
- Protein: 10 grams

What to Use

- 1.50 tsp of baking powder
- 5 Tbsp of butter (melted)
- 2 large eggs
- 0.75 cups of almond flour
- 1.50 tsp of stevia

Baking Instructions

- Preheat oven at 350F. While that is warming up go and grab a muffin top pan. Also, make sure to melt the butter while you're at it.

- Get a medium bowl and place inside the baking powder, almond flour, and stevia.

- Whisk the eggs in a separate large bowl and add them into the first bowl of almond flour, baking powder, and stevia.

- Add the butter in (make sure it is melted first) and then whisk everything together.

- Transfer the batter into the muffin top pan in 6 parts.

- Bake for 15 minutes. Let cool for 5 minutes.

Awesome Keto Flax Buns

This recipe takes about 22 minutes to prepare and bake and makes 3 servings.

This is another recipe that does not contain many ingredients and is quick to the point and is also a good start for beginners. This recipe contains stevia, but any non-sugar-based sweetener will work.

- Calories: 251
- Carbs: 9 grams
- Fat: 22 grams
- Fiber: 8 grams
- Protein: 10 grams

What to Use

- 2 Tbsp of butter
- 0.25 cups of water
- 0.75 cups of flaxseed meal
- 1.5 tsp of stevia
- 1 tsp of salt
- 1.50 tsp of baking powder
- 2 large eggs

Baking Instructions

- Preheat oven at 350F. Go grab a muffin top pan while that is heating up.
- In one large bowl, put the salt, baking powder, stevia, and flaxseed meal. Mix it all together.
- In a second large bowl place inside the eggs, butter, and water. Whisk together.
- Pour the contents from the second bowl (eggs, butter, water) into the first bowl (flaxseed, baking powder, stevia, salt). Combine them and mix them together.
- Transfer the batter into a muffin top pan.
- Bake for 17 minutes. Let cool for 5.

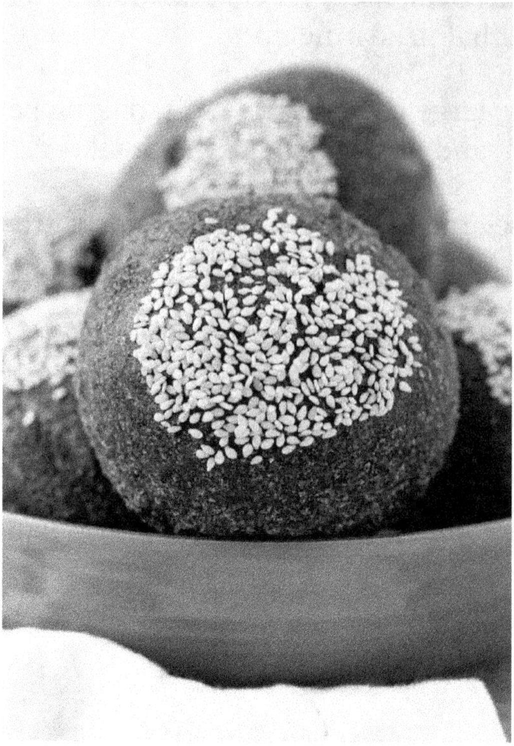

Vegan Keto Bread Buns

This recipe takes about 65 minutes to prepare and bake and makes 6 servings.

This recipe will contain two sets of instructions; 1 for a flax egg and another for the dough, then they will be combined.

- Calories: 229
- Carbs: 25 grams
- Fat: 15 grams
- Fiber: 21 grams
- Protein: 7 grams

What to Use

- 1.25 cups of boiling water (for dough)
- 1.25 tsp of cream of tartar
- 2.50 tsp of baking soda
- 1 tsp of salt
- 0.50 Tbsp of psyllium husk powder
- 0.75 cup of ground flaxseed (for dough)
- 1.25 cup of almond flour
- 0.50 cup of warm water (for flax egg)
- 3 Tbsp of flaxseed (for flax egg)

Baking Instructions

- Preheat oven to 375F. While that is warming up go and grab a baking sheet and line it up with parchment paper.
- Grab a small bowl and place inside it the 0.50 cups of water and the 3 Tbsp of flaxseed. Whisk it together and set to the side. It should settle for 5 minutes. This will make your flax egg.
- Grab a medium bowl and place inside it the almond flour, 0.75 cups of ground flaxseed, psyllium husk powder, salt, baking soda, and cream of tartar. Whisk them all together until they start to form together.
- Start boiling the 1.25 cups of water.
- Place the flax egg in the bowl of almond flour and all his friends. Mix them together (an electric mixer is recommended here) until everything forms well.
- Slowly and carefully pour the boiling water into the dough. Mix everything until it combines.
- Let the dough settle for 5 minutes.
- When ready, break the dough into 6 sections and form them into rolls. Then place the rolls on the parchment paper and baking sheet.
- Bake for 50 minutes.

Keto Cheese and Bacon Cauliflower Buns

This recipe takes about 25 minutes to prepare and bake and makes 12 servings.

- Calories: 346
- Carbs: 8 grams
- Fat: 27 grams
- Fiber: 4 grams
- Protein: 15 grams

What to Use

- 0.75 cups of butter (melted)
- 2 tsp of sea salt
- 4 medium eggs
- 1 tsp of pink Himalayan salt
- 1 tsp of baking powder
- 0.75 cups of almond flour
- 0.75 cups of coconut flour
- 0.625 cups of mozzarella (grated)
- 17.64 ounces of cauliflower (riced)
- 3.53 ounces of bacon (diced)

Baking Instructions

- Preheat oven to 400F. While that is warming up go and grab a baking sheet.
- Fry the bacon for 5 minutes. It should start to give off a light golden appearance.
- Rice the cauliflower using a food processor, unless you bought it already riced.
- Get a large bowl and place every ingredient inside. Mix them all together until they start to combine well.
- Use egg rings to shape the mixture correctly and then place them on the baking sheet.
- Bake for 10 minutes, then take them out and flip them over and bake for another 10 minutes.

Sesame Keto Buns

This recipe takes about 55 minutes to prepare and bake and makes 12 servings.

- Calories: 133
- Carbs: 4 grams
- Fat: 7 grams
- Fiber: 10 grams
- Protein: 7 grams

What to Use

- 8 egg whites
- 1 tbs of baking powder
- 1 tbs of sea salt
- 1 cup of water (boiling)
- 6 Tbsp of psyllium husk powder
- 0.50 cup of pumpkin seeds
- 1 cup of sesame seeds
- 1 cup of coconut flour

Baking Instructions

- Preheat oven to 350F. While that is warming up grab a baking sheet and line it up with parchment paper. Get the water boiling while you're at it.

- Grab a bowl and place inside the coconut flour, sesame seeds, pumpkin seeds, psyllium husk powder, baking powder, and salt. Mix them together. When using the sesame seeds; only use half of the cup. The other half of the cup will be sprinkled atop the buns just before they go into the oven.

- Use a blender to blend the egg whites until they give off a foamy appearance.

- Add the egg whites to the bowl of salt, powders, and seeds.

- Pour the boiling water into the bowl and mix it well.

- Place the buns onto the baking sheet and sprinkle the sesame seeds onto all of them.

- Bake for 50 minutes.

Keto Soul Bread Sesame Rolls

This recipe takes about 32 minutes to prepare and bake and makes 12 servings.

This is an interesting one. It could be placed in many different chapters in this book and can be quite versatile. The "Buns" section is as good as any other for it.

- Calories: 175
- Carbs: 3 grams
- Fat: 15 grams
- Fiber: 0.33 grams
- Protein: 9 grams

What to Use

- 1 cup of sesame seeds
- 0.25 tsp of cream of tartar
- 0.25 tsp of baking soda
- 0.25 tsp of salt
- 0.50 tsp of garlic powder
- 0.50 tsp of xanthan gum
- 1.50 tsp of baking powder
- 1.25 cups of soy protein isolate
- 1 egg white

- 2 eggs
- 2.50 Tbsp of whipping cream
- 2.50 Tbsp of avocado oil
- 3 Tbsp of butter (melted)
- 16 Tbsp of cream cheese (for this recipe it is recommended that the cream cheese is softened).

Baking Instructions

- Preheat oven to 350F. Get a muffin pan ready while it's warming up. Also, make sure the butter is melted.
- Grab a large bowl and place inside it the cream cheese, melted butter, egg white, avocado oil, whipping cream and eggs. Whisk them all together.
- Get a separate large bowl and place inside the cream of tartar, baking soda, salt, garlic powder, baking soda, protein powder and xanthan gum. Whisk them all together.
- Add the bowl of powders and their friends to the bowl of eggs and cream cheese. Fold them in by hand and mix them. Be careful not to over mix this one.
- Use a spoon to transfer the mixture into a muffin top pan.
- Sprinkle the sesame seeds on top of the dough.
- Bake for 25 minutes.

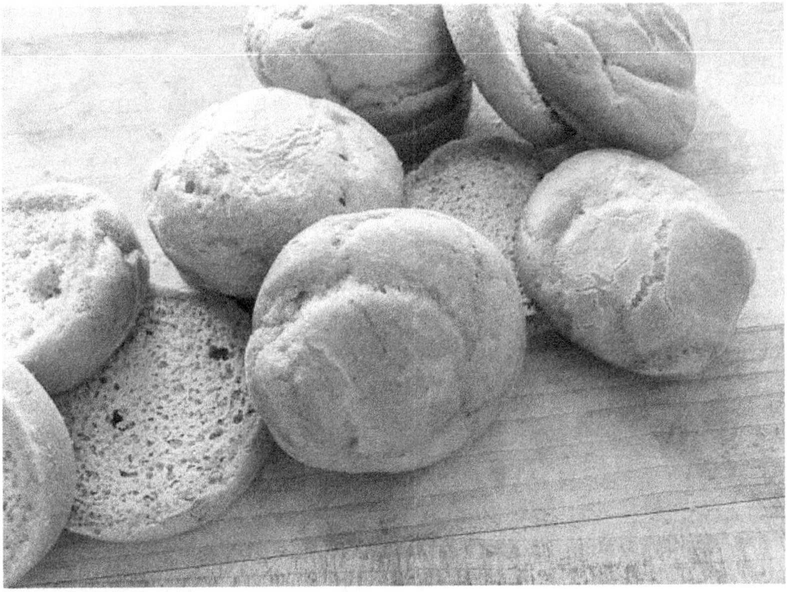

Keto Slider Buns

This recipe takes 27 minutes to prepare and bake and makes 6 servings.

- Calories: 234
- Carbs: 3 grams
- Fat: 15 grams
- Fiber: 2 grams
- Protein: 7 grams

What to Use

- 0.50 tsp of apple cider vinegar
- 0.75 cups of almond flour
- 2 Tbsp of mayonnaise
- 5 Tbsp of avocado oil
- 0.50 tsp of baking soda
- 0.50 tsp of Himalayan salt
- 2 large eggs
- 5 Tbsp of water (warm)
- 1 Tbsp of psyllium husk powder

Baking Instructions

- Preheat oven to 425F.

- Using an immersion blender, place inside the water and psyllium husk powder. Blend together until it takes on a gel-like appearance.

- Add the mayo, avocado oil, baking soda, salt, and eggs into the blender. Blend it all together until it combines.

- Next, add the almond flour, but only a third of the amount. Blend until the almond flour combines, then stop and add another third of the almond flour. Blend it again, then add the final third of the almond flour. Blend it again.

- Add the apple cider vinegar and blend again until there are no lumps left.

- Scoop or spoon the batter into a muffin pan.

- Bake for 22 minutes.

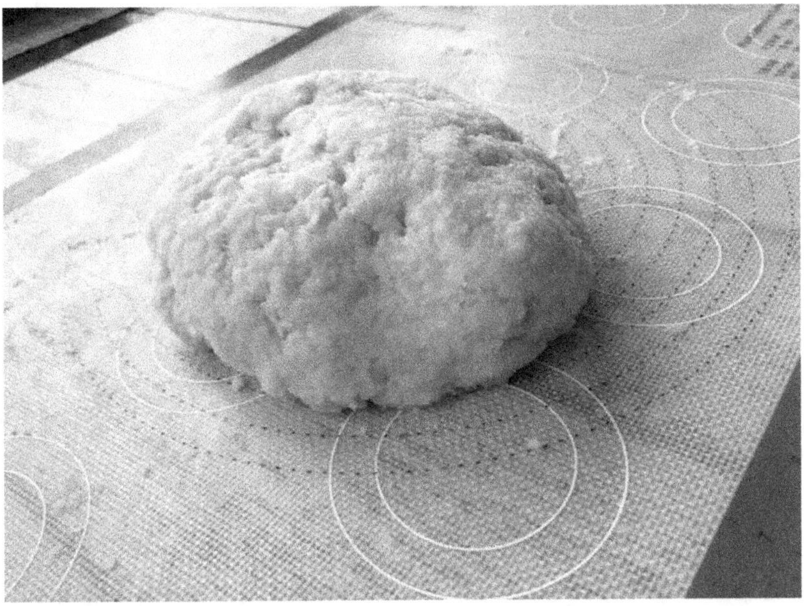

Keto Sweet Hawaiian Buns

This recipe takes 30 minutes to prepare and bake and makes 10 servings.

This recipe contains stevia, but any non-sugar-based sweetener will work.

- Calories: 189
- Carbs: 6 grams
- Fat: 12 grams
- Fiber: 3 grams
- Protein: 16 grams

What to Use

- 1 tsp of ginger paste (fresh is the best)
- 1 tsp of pineapple oil
- 2 eggs
- 0.375 cups of cream cheese
- 3 cups of mozzarella cheese (shredded)
- 0.75 cups of Stevia
- 2 tsp of baking powder
- 1.50 cups of almond flour

Baking Instructions

- Preheat oven to 435F. Grab a baking pan and grease it up.

- Grab a medium bowl and place inside the baking powder, stevia, and almond flour. Mix them together.

- Melt the cream cheese and mozzarella together in a separate bowl. 2 minutes should do the trick. However, stop after only 1 minute and make sure that you stir the cheese. Then heat it for another minute.

- Pour the melted cheese into the bowl of almond flour, stevia, and baking powder.

- Add the eggs, pineapple powder, and ginger paste. Mix everything until it combines well. It will be sticky.

- Cut the dough into 10 parts and roll them into balls.

- Bake for 20 minutes.

Oopsie Baked Keto Buns

This recipe takes about 30 minutes to prepare and bake and makes 4 servings.

- Calories: 80
- Carbs: 4 grams
- Fat: 5 grams
- Fiber: 2 grams
- Protein: 6 grams

What to Use

- 1 Tsp of psyllium husk powder
- 0.25 tsp of baking soda
- 0.1875 of almond flour
- 0.50 cups of avocado puree
- 0.25 tsp of cream of tartar
- 0.25 tsp of sesame seeds
- 4 medium egg whites

Baking Instructions

- Preheat oven to 320F. While that is warming up go and grab a cookie sheet and line it up with parchment paper.
- Place the egg whites in a large bowl and whisk them thoroughly.

- Add the cream of tartar to the eggs and continue to whisk them.

- Add the avocado puree.

- Add the psyllium husk powder, baking soda, and almond flour to the bowl.

- Slowly stir everything together until it begins to combine well. The appearance should contain no lumps, fluffy, and pale greenish in color.

- Divide the batter into 4 buns and place them on the cookie sheet.

- Flatten and round out the buns to form the shape of buns.

- Sprinkle the sesame seeds atop the buns.

- Bake for 15 minutes. Let cool for 10.

Keto Cloud Bread Buns

This recipe takes about 55 minutes to prepare and bake and makes 18 servings.

- Calories: 56
- Carbs: 0.5 grams
- Fat: 3 grams
- Fiber: 0 grams
- Protein: 5 grams

What to Use

- 0.50 cups of soy protein isolate
- 0.25 tsp of salt
- 0.25 tsp of garlic powder
- 0.25 tsp of onion powder
- 0.33 cups of cream cheese
- 0.50 tsp of cream of tartar
- 6 medium eggs

Baking Instructions

- Preheat oven to 300F. While that is warming up go and get a baking tray and grease it up. While you're at it make sure to separate the eggs from the yolk.

- Grab a large bowl and place inside the cream of tartar and the egg whites. Stir them until they mix together.

- Grab another large bowl and place inside the cream cheese, onion powder, garlic powder, salt, soy protein isolate, and egg yolks. Stir until everything blends together well.

- Fold the egg whites into the bowl of the yolk mixture. When folding them in, be careful to not deflate them.

- Transfer the baking mixture onto the baking tray.

- Bake for 50 minutes.

Portabella Mushroom Hamburger Bun

This recipe takes about 25 minutes to prepare and bake and makes 1 serving.

This one may seem a little odd to some people, and it is debatable whether it can be classified as an actual bread, but why not give it a shot? You just may fall in love. It also goes great if you are hankering for a vegan burger. This is also another recipe that is simple, does not contain many ingredients or steps, and is great for beginners.

- Calories: 110
- Carbs: 10 grams
- Fat: 10 grams
- Fiber: 3 grams
- Protein: 5 grams

What to Use

- 2 portabella mushroom caps
- 0.25 tsp of ground black pepper
- 1 tsp of salt
- 1 tsp of oregano
- 1 clove of garlic (minced)
- 0.50 tsp of olive oil

Baking Instructions

- Turn your griddle or grill on and set it to high.
- Grab a large bowl and place inside it the pepper, salt, oregano, minced up garlic, and coconut oil. Let them all mix together until they combine well.
- Take both of your portabella mushroom caps and make sure you clean them well first before doing anything else. Run some cold water over them and scrape out all the gills for each mushroom.
- Add both of the caps of the portabella mushrooms into the bowl of pepper, salt, oregano, garlic, and coconut oil. Let them marinate for about 10 minutes.
- When they are nice and marinated, take both of the caps out of the bowl and place them on the grill alongside whatever meat you may be cooking.
- Cook both of the portabella mushroom caps on the griddle or grill for 10 minutes.
- Serve with your favorite meat or vegan burger.

Chapter 7: The Muffins

If you needed any more proof that the idea of keto baked goods can remain familiar and tasty, then look no further then this chapter. You don't have to give up on muffins just because you are on a keto diet. Check out these recipes to get your mornings started right, or lunch, or dinner. When a muffin is healthy, there is never a bad time for them.

If you would like, you can use muffin paper wraps for all the recipes in this chapter.

Keto Muffin

This recipe takes about 13 minutes to prepare and bake and makes 1 serving.

It is short and to the point, designed to grab a quick muffin if that is all you are in the mood for. It is also a good starter place for beginners.

If wanting more muffins of this variety, then simply multiply the ingredients for how many other muffins you are adding.

- Calories: 113
- Carbs: 5 grams
- Fat: 54
- Fiber: 3 grams
- Protein: 7 grams

What to Use

- 0.125 of salt
- 0.125 baking soda
- 2 tsp of coconut flour
- 1 large egg

Baking Instructions

- Get a pan or ramekin to place the muffin in while baking and preheat the oven to 400F. Grease the baking container with butter or coconut oil.
- Get a small bowl or anything that can fit the 4 ingredients in. Toss in the egg, salt, baking soda, and coconut oil in. Mix and stir them up.
- Transfer the muffin dough into the greased container and bake for 12 minutes.
- Another advantage to this very simple recipe is that you can also heat it in the microwave for only 1 minute if very pressed for time. Of course, this is a matter of preference, but many would agree that food tastes better when cooked in an oven.

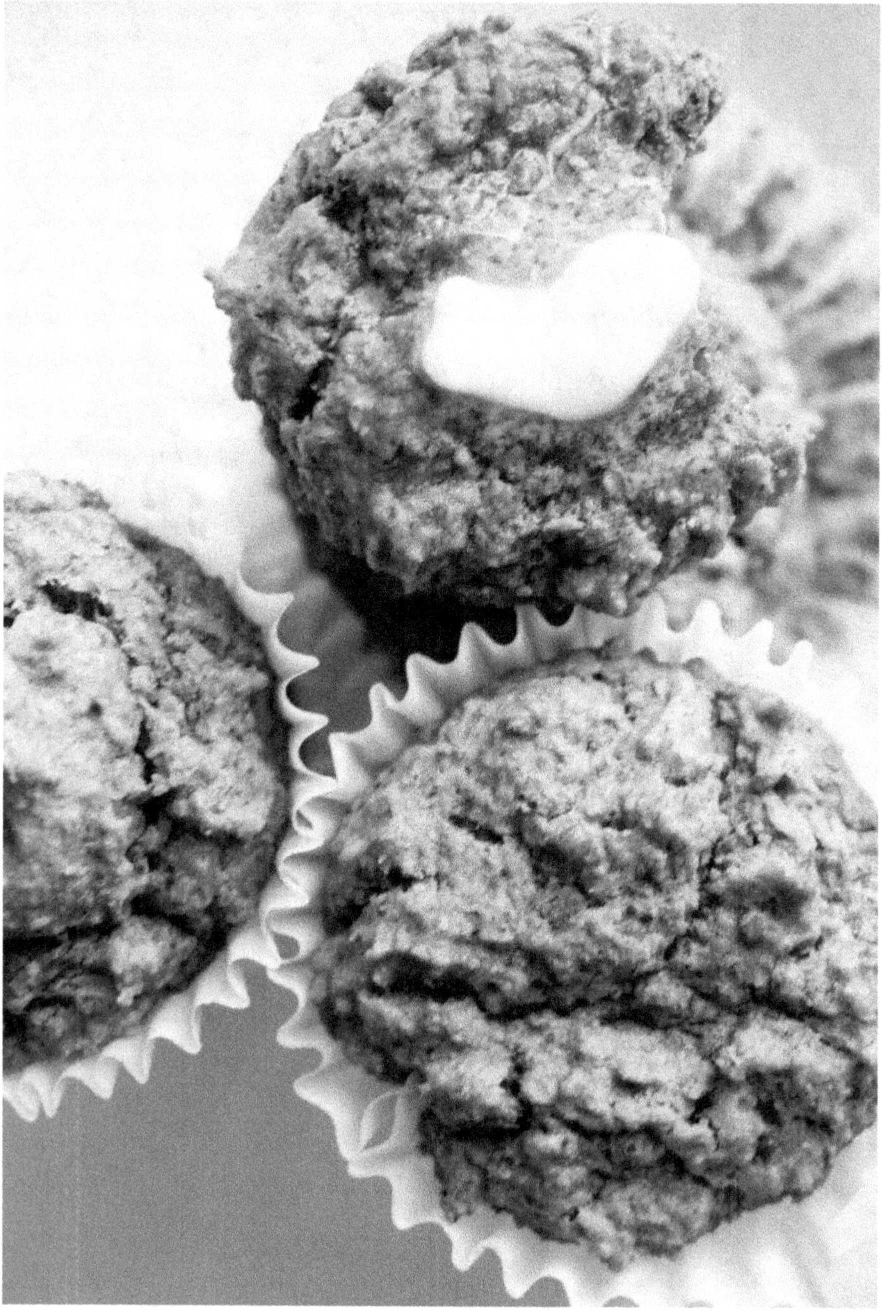

High Fiber Muffins

This recipe takes about 20 minutes to prepare and bake and makes 12 servings

- Calories: 130
- Carbs: 15 grams
- Fat: 11 grams
- Fiber: 16 grams
- Protein: 4 grams

What to Use

- 0.25 tsp of pink Himalayan salt
- 0.50 tsp of vanilla extract
- 2 tsp ground cinnamon
- 0.50 tsp of baking soda
- 1 tsp of baking powder
- 4 Tbsp of erythritol
- 4 Tbsp of butter
- 1 cup of ground flax seed
- 7 Tbsp of heavy whipping cream
- 1 cup oat fiber
- 4 large eggs

Baking Instructions

- Preheat oven to 350F. While that's warming up go and grab a muffin tin and grease it up.

- In the first bowl put in the flaxseed, baking powder, baking soda, cinnamon, salt, and oat fiber.

- In the second bowl place, melt the butter and add the erythritol to it. Mix them both very well.

- Add the vanilla, whipping cream, and eggs to the bowl with butter and erythritol. Mix them all up together.

- Add the contents from the first bowl (flaxseed, baking powder, baking soda, cinnamon, salt, and oat fiber) into the second, wet, bowl. The dough should give off a thick appearance.

- Transfer the dough into the muffin tin.

- Bake for 15 minutes.

Flaxseed Cinnamon Muffins

This recipe takes about 20 minutes to prepare and bake and makes 12 servings.

This recipe contains stevia, but any non-sugar-based sweetener will do.

- Calories: 203
- Carbs: 12 grams
- Fat: 14 grams
- Fiber: 6 grams
- Protein: 6 grams

What to Use

- 2 tsp of vanilla extract
- 0.75 cups of MCT oil
- 0.50 cup of water (water)
- 0.50 tsp of pink Himalayan salt
- 2 Tbsp of ground cinnamon
- 1 Tbsp baking soda
- 0.25 cups of Stevia
- 2 cups of ground flaxseed.
- 5 large eggs

Baking Instructions

- Preheat oven to 350F. While that is warming up grab a muffin tin.
- Grab a large bowl. Place the stevia, cinnamon, salt, baking powder and flax seed inside it. Whisk it all together.
- Get a blender ready. Mix up the eggs, water, vanilla and MCT oil into it. Set the blender to high and blend it all together for 30 seconds.
- Take the blended eggs, MCT, water and vanilla, and pour it into the bowl you used for the cinnamon, salt, baking powder, and stevia Stir it up until it all begins to come together. It should give a fluffy, cloud-like, appearance. Then allow it to sit for 5 minutes.
- After it has settled, grab a spoon and transfer the muffin mixture into a muffin tin until you have filled 12 spots. Remember to not fill the holes all the way because the muffins will rise while baking.
- Bake for 15 minutes. Let cool for 3 minutes.

Cinnamon Seed-plosion Muffins

This recipe takes 35 minutes to prepare and bake and makes 18 servings.

There is a trick to this recipe revolving around the cinnamon. Each muffin gets one teaspoon of cinnamon so you will need 18 teaspoons. It also contains Stevia, but any non-sugar-based sweetener will work. Another trick with the recipe is that, if desired, you can add whatever seeds you want.

- Calories: 181
- Carbs: 5 grams
- Fat: 16 grams
- Fiber: 3 grams
- Protein: 6 grams

What to Use

- 18 tsp of cinnamon (each muffin gets its own teaspoon)
- 2 Tbsp of Stevia
- 0.125 of flaxseed
- 2 Tbsp of chia seeds
- 0.50 cups of unsweetened coconut flakes
- 0.50 cups of pumpkin seeds (shelled)
- 0.50 cups of slivered almonds

- 0.50 cups of walnuts
- 0.25 tsp of sea salt
- 3 tsp of baking powder
- 2 tsp of cinnamon
- 2 tsp of vanilla extract
- 8 Tbsp of coconut oil
- 1 cup of warm water
- 1 cup of almond flour
- 1 cup of golden flaxseed
- 5 large eggs
- If desired, have a separate amount of seeds and nuts of your choice. The amount should be 1 cup of various mixed seeds and nuts.

Baking Instructions

- Preheat oven to 325. While that is warming up go and grab a muffin tin and grease it up.
- Grab a large bowl and place inside it the slivered almonds, coconut flakes, pumpkin seeds and various mixed nuts and seeds (if you decide to use them).
- Then add the almond flour, flax seeds, chia seeds, baking powder, sea salt, cinnamon powder, flax meal, Stevia. Mix everything together.

- Place the water, eggs, and vanilla in a mixer (stand-up mixer is recommended for this) and beat them all tougher.

- Add the beaten eggs, vanilla, and water to the bowl of seeds, nuts, and all their friends. Stir for at least 5 minutes. The batter should combine well and have a thick appearance.

- Transfer 18 muffins into the tin. Each muffin gets a teaspoon of cinnamon individually.

- Bake for 25 minutes. Let cool for 3 minutes.

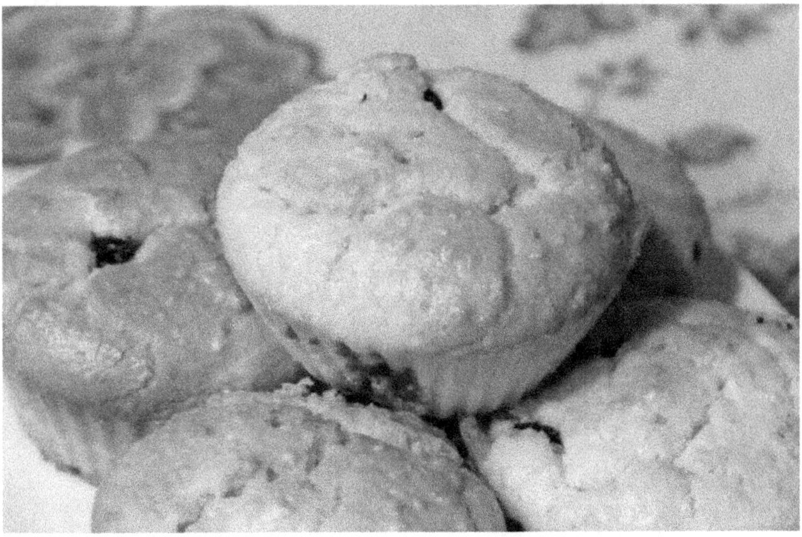

Keto Lemon Blueberry Muffins

This recipe takes 35 about minutes to prepare and bake and makes 12 servings. Stevia is in this recipe, but any non-sugar-based sweetener will work.

- Calories: 223
- Carb: 5 grams
- Fat: 2 grams
- Fiber: 3 grams
- Protein: 5 grams

What to Use

- 0.25 tsp lemon zest
- 0.50 tsp lemon extract
- 0.50 cups of blueberries (the fresher, the better)
- 1 tsp of baking soda
- 0.50 tsp of stevia
- 0.25 cups of butter
- 2 cups of almond flour
- 1 cup of heavy whipping cream
- 2 large eggs

Baking Instructions

- Preheat oven to 350F. While the oven is warming up go grab a muffin tin and grease it up. Also, make sure to melt the butter and zest the lemon.

- Put both eggs in a large bowl and mix them up together.

- Add the stevia, butter, baking soda, blueberries, lemon extract, lemon zest, almond flour, and whipping cream into the bowl with the eggs. Mix them up till they take form together.

- Pour 12 muffins into a baking pan.

- Bake for 30 minutes.

Keto Blueberry Muffins

This recipe takes about 25 minutes to prepare and bake and makes 12 servings.

- Calories: 217
- Carbs: 6 grams
- Fat: 19 grams
- Fiber: 3 grams
- Protein: 7 grams

What to Use

- 0.75 cups of blueberries
- 0.50 tsp of vanilla extract
- 0.50 cups of almond milk, unsweetened
- 8 Tbsp of coconut oil (this should be melted before adding it)
- 1.5 tsp of baking powder
- 6 Tbsp of erythritol
- 2.50 cups of almond flour
- 3 large eggs

Baking Instructions

- Preheat oven to 350F. Melt the coconut oil while preheating. Grab a muffin pan and line it up with parchment paper.

- In a large bowl, you will add the baking powder, erythritol, and almond flour. Stir and mix them all up.
- Then, to the same bowl add the eggs, almond milk, vanilla extract, and coconut oil (melted).
- Then add the blueberries to the mixture, but make sure to carefully fold them when adding them.
- Place the batter from the bowl into the muffin pan.
- Bake for 20 minutes.

Low Carb Bacon and Broccoli Muffins

This recipe takes about 25 minutes to prepare and bake and makes 12 servings.

- Calories: 105
- Carbs: 3 grams
- Fat: grams
- Fiber: 1 gram
- Protein: 8 grams

What to Use

- 12 slices of bacon (thinly sliced)
- 0.50 Tbsp of olive oil
- 4 ounces of broccoli
- 0.50 cups of cheddar cheese (shredded)
- 0.50 cups of heavy cream
- 4 large egg whites
- 6 large eggs

Baking Instructions

- Preheat oven to 350F. Get a baking pan out while it's preheating and grease it up.
- Take the bacon slices and place them in the baking pan after greasing the pan. You will want to roll the bacon into circular shapes, so it wraps

around the edges where the muffins will go before being placed in the oven.

- In one large bowl place the egg whites, eggs, and heavy cream. Mix them together.

- Heat up the broccoli in the microwave. Then place the broccoli along with the bacon in the baking pan.

- Top the broccoli and bacon with the cheddar cheese.

- Pour the muffin batter into the pan with the cheese, bacon, and broccoli. If you want more cheese, this is a good time to sprinkle a little bit more onto the muffins before going in the oven.

- Bake for 20 minutes.

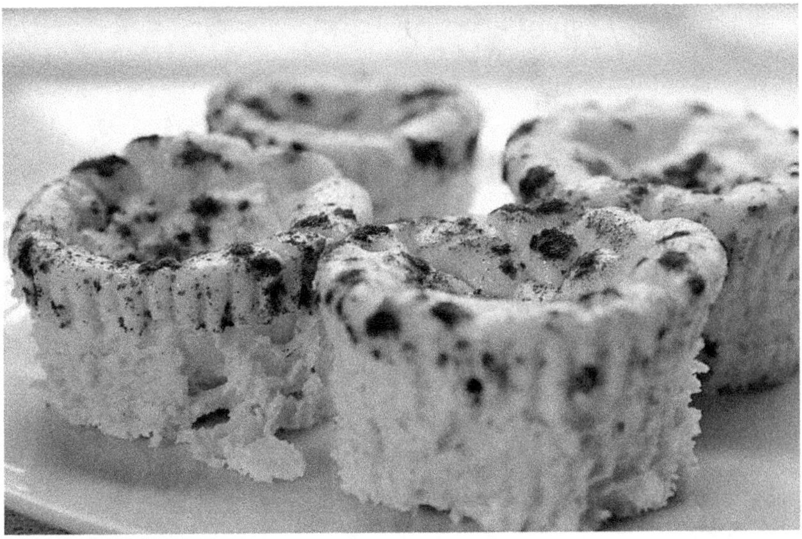

Cream Cheese Muffins

This recipe takes about 30 minutes to prepare and bake and makes 10 servings.

- Calories: 63
- Carbs: 1 gram
- Fat: 6 grams
- Fiber: 0 grams
- Protein: 2 grams

What to Use

- 1 tsp of cinnamon
- 0.50 tsp of vanilla extract
- 6 Tbsp of erythritol
- 2 medium eggs
- 16 tsp of cream cheese

Baking Instructions

- Preheat oven to 350F. While that is warming up go and grab a muffin tin.
- Go get a large bowl and add the vanilla, eggs, erythritol, and cream cheese. Mix them together until they give off a soft appearance.
- Place the mixture into a muffin tin. Add the cinnamon atop the mixture.

- Bake for 20 minutes.

Pumpkin Cream Cheese Muffins

This recipe takes about 30 minutes to prepare and makes 20 servings.

There are two sets of instructions for this one. One for the muffins, and another for the filling.

- Calories: 147
- Carbs: 3 grams
- Fat: 13 grams
- Fiber: 0.3 grams
- Protein: 3 grams

What to Use for the muffins

- 1.50 tsp of baking powder
- 0.50 tsp of salt
- 0.125 cups of coconut flour
- 1.50 tsp of vanilla extract
- 6 Tbsp of stevia
- 2 Tbsp of sour cream
- 1 cup of pumpkin pie spice
- 1 cup of pumpkin puree
- 2 Tbsp of butter

- 6 Tbsp of coconut oil (this should be melted ahead of time)
- 6 medium eggs

What to Use for the filling

- 0.50 tsp of vanilla extract
- 05 Tbsp of stevia
- 1 Tbsp of heavy whipping cream
- 0.375 cups of cream cheese.

Baking Instructions

- Preheat oven to 350F. While that is warming up go and grab a muffin tin and grease it up. Also, make sure to melt both the butter and coconut oil.
- Grab a large bowl and add the eggs, pumpkin pie spice, pumpkin puree, sour cream, vanilla extract, and stevia. Beat them all together until they mix well.
- In a separate medium bowl, you will want to add the baking powder, salt, and coconut flour.
- Pour the mixture of baking powder, salt, and coconut flour into the first bowl with the eggs, pumpkin ingredients, and everything else. Mix them all together well.
- Transfer the muffin batter into the tin. Add the cream cheese (0.50 tsp each) on top.

- Use a spoon, a toothpick, or anything small, to swirl the muffin batter and cream cheese.

- Bake for 25 minutes.

Super Cheesy Keto Garlic Bread Muffins

This recipe takes about 45 minutes to prepare and bake and makes 6 servings.

There are two sets of directions listed here. One for the muffins. The other for the garlic topping.

- Calories: 270
- Carbs: 8 grams
- Fat: 23 grams
- Fiber: 5 grams
- Protein: 8 grams

What to Use for the Garlic Topping

- 0.50 tsp of salt
- 0.50 tsp of garlic powder
- 2 tsp of basil (dried)
- 2 Tbsp of butter (melted)

What to Use for the Muffins

- 0.75 cups of cheddar cheese (grated)
- 0.375 cups of water (warm)
- 2 medium egg yolks
- 1 tsp of apple cider vinegar
- 0.25 cups of butter (melted)

- 2 medium egg whites
- 0.50 tsp of garlic powder
- 0.50 tsp of salt
- 0.50 tsp of baking powder
- 0.50 tsp of baking soda
- 0.50 tsp of xanthan gum
- 2 Tbsp of psyllium husk powder
- 0.1875 cups of coconut flour
- 1 cup of almond flour

Baking Instructions for the Garlic Topping

- Grab a bowl and place inside the butter (melted), basil, salt, and garlic powder. Mix them all together and set aside for later use.

Baking Instructions for the Muffins

- Preheat oven to 350F. While that is warming up go and grab a muffin tray and grease it up. Also, beat the eggs and set aside for later.

- Grab a medium bowl and place inside it the garlic powder, salt, baking soda, baking powder, xanthan gum, psyllium husk powder, almond flour, and coconut flour. Whisk them all together.

- Grab another large bowl and place inside the butter (0.25 cups). Make sure the butter is melted first. Use a mixer (an electric one is recommended) for 1 minute to cream the butter.

- Add the egg yolks and apple cider vinegar to the bowl of butter. Beat everything together until they blend well.

- Take the contents from the medium bowl (almond flour, coconut flour, and all their friends) and pour half of it in. Then pour the water in and beat the mixture together. Then pour in the rest of the contents from the medium bowl (almond flour, coconut flour) and beat it until it blends.

- Add the cheddar cheese. Then fold in the egg whites. When folding them in, it is recommended to do so gently as to not deflate them. Mix it up a little more.

- Transfer the batter with a spoon into the muffin tray. If need be, even out the tops.

- Bake for 20 minutes.

- Stop baking them and brush with the garlic topping. When brushing the muffin tops, be gentle as to not disturb the integrity of the dough.

- Bake for another 10 minutes. Allow to cool for 15 minutes.

Chapter 8: The Crackers

Here they are, the crackers. Consider this chapter to be another reason why going keto can be a tasty lifestyle to transform into. Let's face it, we all like a quick snack to have on the go or at home and with these keto crackers, there is absolutely no excuse to ever go for a candy bar or donut ever again. They can all be eaten for standalone snacking or topped with whatever your heart may desire at that moment (as long as the toppings are also keto friendly). Get ready to dive into a new way of thinking about and enjoying crackers!

An extra thing to note about baking the crackers is that the serving sizes can vary by a substantial margin. This is all due to personal preference. Some people like crackers to be square, while others prefer rectangles, and some may want them to be triangular. Since the shapes can vary, so can the sizes and that will affect the serving amounts. Each recipe listed here will have a recommended shape and serving size, but you are free to experiment at your own discretion.

Easy Keto Crackers

This recipe takes about 22 minutes to prepare and bake and makes 5 servings. There are only three ingredients, thus the word "Easy" in the name.

- Calories: 226
- Carbs: 8 grams
- Fat: 19 grams
- Fiber: 4 grams
- Protein: 9 grams

What to Use

- 1 large egg
- 0.50 tsp of sea salt
- 2 cups of almond flour

Baking Instructions

- Preheat oven to 350F. While that is warming up grab a baking sheet and line it up with parchment paper.
- Go get a large bowl and combine the almond flour with the salt.
- Beat the egg separately before adding it to the almond flour and salt.
- Add the egg to the bowl and mix them all together until they combine well. If desired and in a rush, you may also use a food processor.

- Place the dough on the baking sheet and roll them into rectangle shapes. If needed, rip or cut the dough after rolling them (if there are excess edges complicating the shape).

- Bake for 12 minutes.

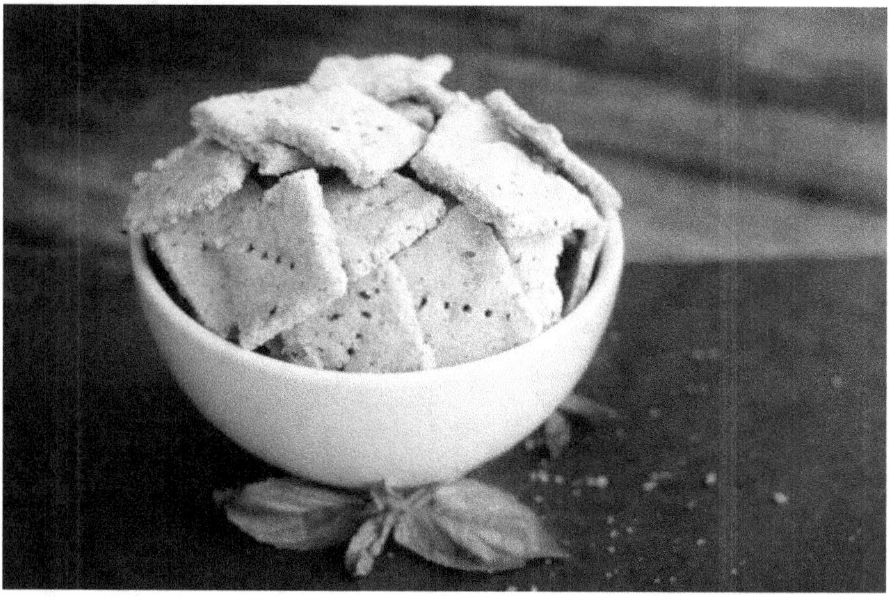

Keto Pesto Crackers

This recipe takes about 25 minutes to prepare and bake and makes 6 servings.

- Calories: 204
- Carbs: 6 grams
- Fat: 19 grams
- Fiber: 2 grams
- Protein: 5 grams

What to Use

- 3 Tbsp of butter
- 2 Tbsp of basil pesto
- 1 clove of garlic (pressed)
- 0.16 tsp of cayenne pepper
- 0.25 tsp of dried basil
- 0.50 tsp of baking powder
- 0.50 tsp of salt
- 0.25 tsp of ground black pepper
- 1.25 cups of almond flour

Baking Instructions

- Preheat oven to 325F. While that is warming up grab a cookie sheet and line it up with parchment paper.

- Grab a medium bowl and place inside it the baking powder, salt, pepper, and almond flour. Whisk them all together.
- Add the garlic, cayenne pepper, and basil. Stir everything until it combines well.
- Add the pesto to the mix and whisk it in with everything else.
- Add the butter into the mixture, and stir it till the mixture takes the form of a ball.
- Place the dough onto the baking sheet.
- Bake for 17 minutes. When it is done, cut the dough into rectangular cracker shaped pieces.

Low Carb Fathead Keto Crackers

This recipe takes about 20 minutes to prepare and bake and makes 6 servings.

- Calories: 203
- Carbs: 4 grams
- Fat: 17 grams
- Fiber: 2 grams
- Protein: 11 grams

What to Use

- 1 medium egg
- 2 Tbsp of cream cheese
- 0.75 cups of almond flour
- 0.50 tsp of salt
- 0.50 cups of mozzarella cheese (shredded)

Baking Instructions

- Preheat oven to 425F. Grab a baking sheet while it is warming up.
- Get a large bowl for the mozzarella and almond flour. Mix the two of them together, then add the cream cheese. Heat them up in the microwave for 1 minute.
- Add the salt and egg. Gently mix them together.

- Place the dough on the baking sheet and use a rolling pin to level them until they are thin. Cut the dough into rectangular, cracker shaped pieces.
- Bake for 5 minutes, then flip them over and bake for another 5 minutes, so each side is evened out.

Low Carb Keto Cheese Crackers

This recipe takes about 20 minutes to prepare and bake and makes 10 servings.

- Calories: 94
- Carbs: 3 grams
- Fat: 8 grams
- Fiber: 1 gram
- Protein: 4 grams

What to Use

- 1 tsp of rosemary
- 0.50 tsp of sea salt
- 1 medium egg
- 4 Tbsp of cream cheese
- 1 cup of almond flour
- 2 cups of parmesan cheese

What to Use

- Preheat oven to 450F. While that is warming up get a baking sheet and line it with parchment paper.
- Grab a bowl and place inside it the cream cheese, parmesan, and almond flour. Heat it the microwave

for 1 minute (keep in mind that microwave times may vary).

- Stir the mixture until everything forms together well. Allow it to cool for 3 minutes before moving onto next step.

- When it has cooled, add the rosemary, salt, and egg. Mix it all together. If it becomes too hard and difficult to mix, then microwave for another 20 seconds.

- Transfer the dough onto the baking sheet and roll it until it has a thin layer. Cut the crackers into small squares.

- Bake for 6 minutes, then take them out and flip them over and bake for another 6 minutes to make sure everything bakes evenly. Allow to cool for 5 minutes.

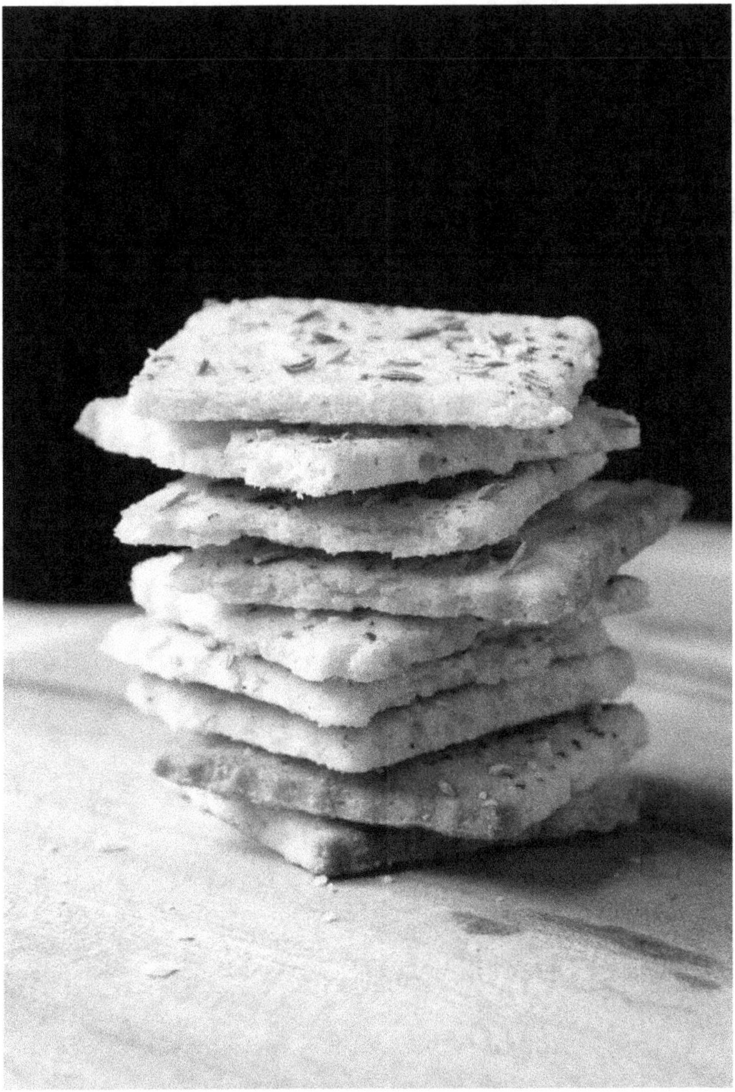

Flakey Cream Cheese Keto Crackers

This recipe takes about 95 minutes to prepare and bake and makes 8 servings.

- Calories: 189
- Carbs: 4 grams
- Fat: 17 grams
- Fiber: 2 grams
- Protein: 3 grams

What to Use

- 0.50 cups of caraway seeds
- 0.50 cups of garlic powder
- 2 medium egg (one of them will be used for egg wash, the other for the yolk)
- 2 tsp of apple cider vinegar
- 0.25 cups of cream cheese
- 1.25 cups of cups of butter
- 0.50 tsp of salt
- 0.50 tsp of xanthan gum
- 03125 cups of coconut flour
- 1 cup of almond flour

Baking Instructions

- Grab a food processor and place inside it the salt, xanthan gum, coconut flour, and almond flour. Pulse 5-6 times or until everything has combined together evenly.

- Add the cream cheese and butter into the food processor. Pulse it for a few seconds, but make sure to stop before the dough takes the form of a ball. You are looking for the dough to have a coarse appearance.

- Add the egg yolk to the food processor.

- Grab some cling film and wrap the dough into a round shape.

- Place it in the refrigerator for one hour.

- When the dough is ready to come out of the fridge, grab a baking sheet and line it up with parchment paper.

- Roll the dough onto parchment paper and cut it into rectangular shapes. Then place it back in the fridge for another 10 minutes. Preheat the oven to 350F while waiting.

- When ready, take the dough out of the fridge and place the parchment paper and dough onto a baking sheet.

- Brush the dough with the egg wash.

- Sprinkle the dough with the caraway seeds and garlic powder.

- Bake for 20 minutes.

Keto Almond Flour Crackers

This recipe takes about 30 minutes to prepare and bake and makes 24 servings.

- Calories: 140
- Carbs: 4 grams
- Fat: 13 grams
- Fiber: 2 grams
- Protein: 6 grams

What to Use

- 1.75 cups of blanched almond flour (ground)
- 0.50 tsp of black pepper
- 0.25 tsp of salt
- 1 large egg

Baking Instructions

- Preheat oven to 350F. While that is warming up grab a baking sheet and lime it up with some parchment paper.
- Grab a medium bowl and place inside it the salt, pepper, and egg. Whisk them all together.
- Add the almond flour and whisk it in.
- Put the dough on the baking sheet and roll them into a thin layer.

- Cut the crackers into small square shapes.
- Bake for 16 minutes.

Keto Heavy Seed Crackers

This recipe takes about 60 minutes to prepare and bake and makes 30 servings.

- Calories: 61
- Carbs: 3 grams
- Fat: 6 grams
- Fiber: 1 gram
- Protein: 2 grams

What to Use

- 1 cup of water (boiling)
- 4 Tbsp of coconut oil (melted)
- 1 tsp of salt
- 1 Tbsp of psyllium husk powder
- 0.75 cups of sesame seeds
- 0.75 cups of chia seeds
- 0.75 cups of pumpkin seeds
- 0.75 cups of sunflower seeds
- 0.75 cups of almond flour

Baking Instructions

- Preheat oven to 300F. Grab a baking sheet and line it up with some parchment paper while the oven warms up. Also get the water boiling while you're at it.

- Grab a large bowl and place inside it the almond flour, sunflower seeds, pumpkin seeds, chia seeds, sesame seeds, psyllium husk powder, and salt. Mix them all together.

- Add the coconut oil and water. The water should be boiling so make sure to pour it in slowly and carefully.

- Place the dough onto the baking sheet and roll it into a thin layer.

- Bake for 45 minutes. Using the lower rack is recommended. Also, seeds can be heat sensitive when baking, and there are a lot of them in this recipe so check every few minutes to make sure seeds aren't popping out all over the place.

- Leave it in the oven to dry for 15 minutes.

- When ready, break the crackers into squares or rectangles.

Easy Coconut Keto Cheese Crackers

This recipe takes about 25 minutes to prepare and bake and makes 30 servings.

With a food processor on hand, this is a very simple recipe to bake.

- Calories: 181
- Carbs: 4 grams
- Fat: 14 grams
- Fiber: 8 grams
- Protein: 8 grams

What to Use

- 0.25 tsp of garlic powder
- 0.25 tsp of onion powder
- 0.25 tsp of paprika
- 0.25 tsp of salt
- 0.50 cups of almond flour
- 2 Tbsp of butter
- 1 medium egg
- 0.25 cups of cream cheese
- 2 cups of cheddar jack cheese (shredded)

Baking Instructions

- Preheat oven to 350F. While it is warming up go grab a baking sheet and line it with parchment paper.
- Get a food processor ready and place inside the cream cheese, cheddar, egg, butter, almond flour, salt, paprika, onion powder, garlic powder. Process everything until it combines well.
- Transfer the dough onto the baking sheet and roll it into a thin layer.
- Cut the dough into tiny square shapes.
- Bake for 20 minutes.

Lemon Peppered Parmesan Cheese Crackers

This recipe takes about 60 minutes to prepare and bake and makes 10 servings.

- Calories: 174
- Carbs: 5 grams
- Fat: 14 grams
- Fiber: 2 grams
- Protein: 9 grams

What to Use

- 1 Tbsp of lemon pepper
- 1 Tbsp of olive oil
- 2 large eggs
- 0.25 tsp of granulated onion
- 0.25 tsp of granulated garlic
- 0.25 tsp of baking soda
- 0.25 cups of red mill nutritional yeast
- 0.75 cups of parmesan cheese (grated)
- 2 cups of almond flour

Baking Instructions

- Preheat oven to 350F. While that is heating up go and grab a baking pan and line it with parchment paper.

- Get a medium bowl and place inside the onion, garlic, baking soda, lemon pepper, yeast, parmesan cheese, and almond flour. Whisk them thoroughly. There should be no clumps left after whisking.

- Get a small bowl and place the eggs, and olive oil inside. Whisk them together.

- Add the eggs and olive oil to the first bowl of cheese, lemon pepper, and all their friends. Stir them and form them into a ball of dough.

- Place the dough on the baking sheet and use your hands to flatten it until it is thin.

- Cut the dough into tiny square shapes.

- Bake for 15 minutes, let cool for 5. Break the dough up and spread them evenly and then bake for another 10 minutes.

Keto Graham Crackers

This recipe takes about 85 minutes to prepare and bake and makes 10 servings.

- Calories: 156
- Carbs: 6 grams
- Fat: 14 grams
- Fiber: 3 grams
- Protein: 5 grams

What to Use

- 1 tsp of vanilla extract
- 2 Tbsp of butter (melted)
- 1 large egg
- 0.16 tsp of salt
- 1 tsp of baking powder
- 2 tsp of cinnamon
- 10 tsp of stevia
- 2 cups of almond flour

Baking Instructions

- Preheat oven to 300F. While that is warming up grab a baking sheet and line it with parchment paper. Melt the butter while you're at it.

- Get a large bowl and place inside it the stevia, salt, baking powder cinnamon, and almond flour. Whisk everything together.
- Stir in the vanilla extract, butter, and egg. Keep stirring it until everything forms together nicely.
- Transfer the dough onto the baking sheet and use a rolling pin to roll it until it is smooth.
- Bake for 20 minutes. Let them cool for 30 minutes, break them up, and bake for another 30 minutes.

Rosemary and Raisin Crackers

This recipe takes about 40 minutes to prepare and bake and makes 14 servings.

This recipe contains stevia, but any non-sugar-based sweetener will work.

- Calories: 154
- Carbs: 6 grams
- Fat: 13 grams
- Fiber: 3 grams
- Protein: 6 grams

What to Use

- 1 tsp of rosemary (chopped up)
- 3 Tbsp of raisins
- 1 tsp of salt
- 2 large eggs
- 2 cups of almond flour (blanched)

Baking Instructions

- Preheat oven to 350F. While that is warming up grab a baking sheet and line it with parchment paper.
- Grab a medium bowl and place inside it the salt and almond flour.

- Take the raisins and cut them in half. Then add them to the bowl.
- Add the rosemary. Mix everything together.
- Beat the eggs and add them to the bowl. Stir everything together.
- Separate the dough into 6 pieces and place them on the baking sheet. Roll them with a rolling pin until they are flat and thin.
- Cut the dough into rectangular shapes.
- Bake for 30 minutes.

Keto Fun Crackers

This recipe takes about 35 minutes to prepare and bake and makes 12 servings.

- Calories: 116
- Carbs: 2 grams
- Fat: 11 grams
- Fiber: 1 grams
- Protein: 2 grams

What to Use

- 2 cups of almond flour (blanched)
- 0.50 tsp of sea salt
- 1 tsp of vanilla extract

- 0.25 tsp of baking powder
- 0.50 cups of stevia
- 4 Tbsp of cream cheese
- 0.25 cups of butter

Baking Instructions

- Preheat oven to 300F. While that is warming up go and grab a baking sheet and line it up with parchment paper.
- Get a large bowl and place inside it the butter and cream cheese. Stir it until it mixes together.
- Add the salt, vanilla extract, baking powder, and stevia. Stir it all up.
- Add the almond flour and stir it up.
- Chill for 20 minutes.
- When ready, place the chilled dough on the baking sheet. Flatten it out with a rolling pin until it is nice and thin. If it solidified too much while chilling, then give it a few minutes to thaw.
- Cut the dough into rectangular shapes.
- Bake for 15 minutes.

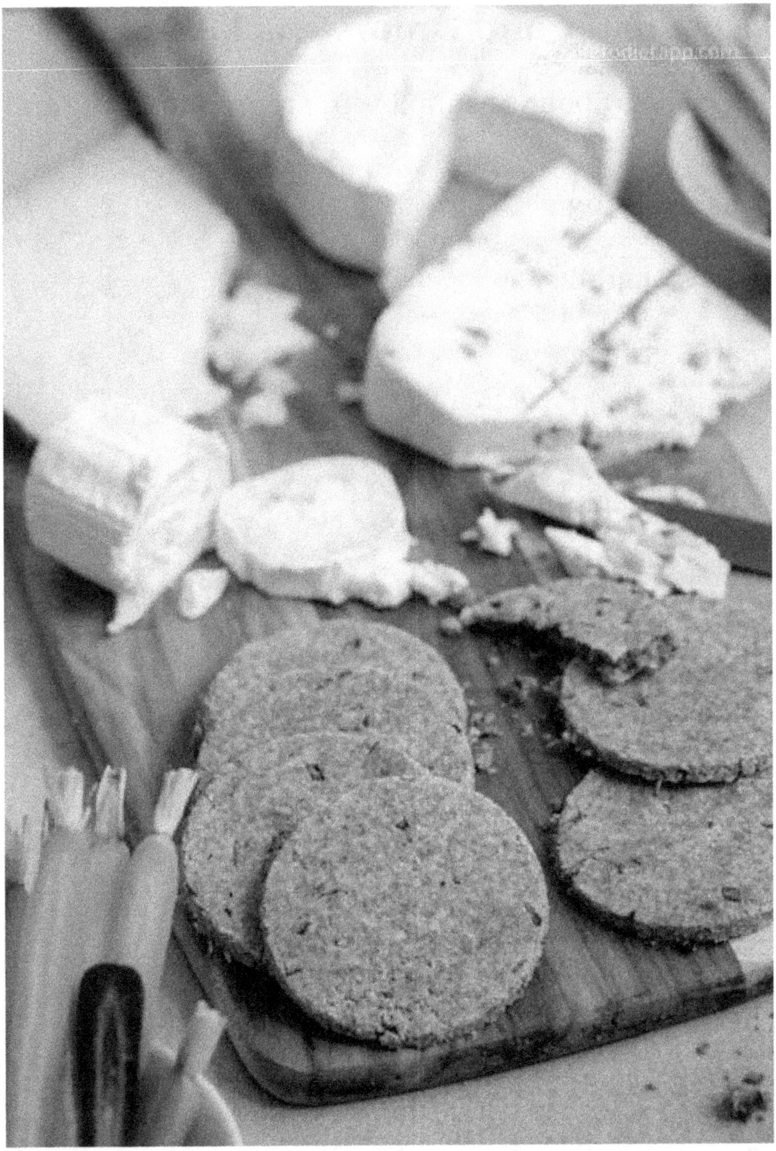

Keto Rosemary and Onion Crackers

This recipe takes about 22 minutes to prepare and bake and makes 4 servings.

- Calories: 103
- Carbs: 4 grams
- Fat: 8 grams
- Fiber: 3 grams
- Protein: 4 grams

What to Use

- 0.75 tsp of black pepper
- 0.75 of pink Himalayan salt
- 1 large egg
- 1 Tbsp of olive oil
- 1 tsp of baking soda
- 0.50 tsp of onion powder
- 2 Tbsp of rosemary (chopped)
- 0.50 cup of flaxseed
- 1 cup of almond (ground)

Baking Instructions

- Preheat oven to 350F. While that is warming up go and grab a baking sheet and line it up with parchment paper.

- Grab a large bowl and place inside it the pepper, salt, baking soda, onion powder, rosemary (make sure it is chopped up first), flaxseed, and almonds. Mix them all up together.

- Grab a separate medium bowl and place inside it the olive oil and egg. Whisk them together until they take form.

- Pour the contents from the egg and olive oil into the first bowl of the rosemary and all its buddies. Mix them together until they combine well

- Transfer the ball onto the baking sheet after rolling it into the shape of a ball.

- Roll the ball of dough flat until it is nice and thin. Use either your hands or a rolling pin.

- The recommended shape for these crackers is circular, so use a cookie cutter to press and cut them into a circle.

- Bake for 15 minutes.

Keto Party Crackers

This recipe takes about 60 minutes to prepare and bake and makes 8 servings.

- Calories: 168
- Carbs: 6 grams
- Fat: 13 grams
- Fiber: 5 grams
- Protein: 8 grams

What to Use

- 1 cup of water (warm)
- 0.25 tsp of black pepper
- 1 tsp of sea salt
- 1 cup of parmesan cheese (grated)
- 1 Tbsp of psyllium husk powder
- 0.50 cup of flaxseed meal
- 1 cup of almond flour

Baking Instructions

- Preheat oven to 325F. While that is warming up go and grab a baking pan and line it with parchment paper.

- Grab a large bowl and place inside it the pepper, salt, psyllium husk powder, flaxseed meal, and almond flour. Mix it all together.

- Add the parmesan cheese to the bowl and mix it together with everything else.

- Add the water. Mix it with everything else already in the bowl. Then let it sit for 10 minutes.

- When ready, divide the dough in half. Place one half on the baking sheet and roll it flat. Then place down the other half of the dough and roll that one flat as well. When rolling them, aim to form them into rectangular shapes.

- Cut both halves of the dough into 16 pieces (32 total).

- Bake for 45 minutes.

Sunny Keto Crackers

This recipe takes 50 minutes to prepare and bake and makes 30 servings.

- Calories: 75
- Carbs: 4 grams
- Fat: 6 grams
- Fiber: 3 grams
- Protein: 2 grams

What to Use

- 1.50 cups of water (warm)
- 1 tsp of salt
- 4 Tbsp of psyllium husk powder
- 0.50 cups of sunflower seeds
- 0.25 cups of sunflower almonds
- 1.50 cup of sesame seeds

Baking Instructions

- Preheat oven to 350F. While that is warming up go and get a baking sheet and line it with parchment paper.
- Grab a large bowl and place inside it the sesame seeds, sunflower almonds, sunflower seeds, psyllium husk powder, and salt. Mix them all together well.

- Add the water. Stir everything together and then let it sit for 10 minutes. It will swell up.
- When ready, break the dough in half and place one half on the baking sheet. Roll it flat with a rolling pin. Then cut the dough into tiny squares.
- Repeat this for the other half of the dough as well.
- Bake for 15 minutes. Take it out and cut the dough to separate the crackers, flip them over, and bake the opposite side for another 15 minutes.

Pumpkin Spice Keto Crackers

This recipe takes about 40 minutes to prepare and bake and makes 20 servings.

- Calories: 106
- Carbs: 60 grams
- Fat: 81 grams
- Fiber: 12 grams
- Protein: 13 grams

What to Use

- 1.75 cups of water (warm)
- 3 Tbsp of coconut oil (melted)
- 1 tsp of salt
- 1 Tbsp of psyllium husk powder
- 0.75 cups of sesame seeds
- 0.75 cups of flaxseed
- 2 Tbsp of pumpkin pie spice
- 0.75 cups of coconut flour

Baking Instructions

- Preheat oven to 300F. While that is warming up get a baking sheet and line it with parchment paper. Also, make sure to melt the coconut oil.

- Get a large bowl and place inside it the coconut flour, pumpkin pie spice, flaxseed, sesame seeds, psyllium husk powder, and salt. Mix everything together till it blends well.

- Add the water and coconut oil. Stir them till they mix well. Let it sit for 3 minutes.

- Bake for 30 minutes. Let it cool for 5 minutes. Cut the crackers into tiny squares.

Grain-Free Cheesy Spinach Crackers

This recipe takes about 70 minutes to prepare and bake and makes 16 servings.

- Calories: 126
- Carbs: 4 grams
- Fat: 11 grams
- Fiber: 3 grams
- Protein: 5 grams

What to Use

- 0.50 tsp of pink Himalayan salt
- 0.50 cups of parmesan cheese (grated)
- 0.50 tsp of dried chili peppers (flaked)
- 0.50 tsp of cumin (ground)
- 0.25 cups of butter
- 0.50 cups of flax meal

- 0.25 cups of coconut flour
- 1.50 cups of almond flour
- 1 cup of spinach (fresh is the best)
- Water (warm, used for the saucepan)
- 2 cups of water (cold)

Baking Instructions

- Grab a saucepan and fill it with water. Turn the stovetop on to high. Make sure to wait for the water to start boiling over.
- When the water is boiling, place the spinach in the pan. Cook for 1 minute.
- When the spinach is ready, take it out of the saucepan and place it in a large bowl filled with cold water. Give it a few seconds to cool off.
- Pick up the spinach and squeeze, strain, the water out of the leaves.
- Grab a blender and place the spinach inside. Blend for 1 minute until it gives off a smooth appearance. Set it to the side for later use.
- Grab another large bowl and place inside it the parmesan cheese, salt, chili flakes, cumin, flax meal, coconut flour, and almond flour. Mix everything together until they blend well.

- Place the blended spinach in the bowl of parmesan cheese and all his friends. Then add the butter.

- Mix everything together until it combines well. Using your own hands is recommended for mixing and blending the spinach.

- Grab a piece of foil and wrap up the dough. Place it in the fridge for 45 minutes.

- Preheat the oven to 400 F. While that is warming up go and grab a baking tray and place parchment paper over it.

- When ready, place the spinach onto the baking sheet. Use a rolling pin to flatten the spinach.

- Use a pizza cutter to cut the dough of spinach into 16 separate pieces.

- Bake for 20 minutes.

Chapter 9: Do It Yourself Breadsticks

Let's be honest here, how many times have you decided to go out to a restaurant, ordered a pizza, or not cooked at home just to get the breadsticks? We are all guilty of this. Using these recipes, you won't have those cravings to run out just to get what most restaurants consider to be appetizers anymore. Admittedly there are not many recipes listed in this chapter. The reason why is because most breadstick recipes are more or less the same thing, and when looking over the keto version of breadsticks, there are unfortunately even fewer options to choose from. Even so, you should give these recipes a look over as there you may find a few nice surprises.

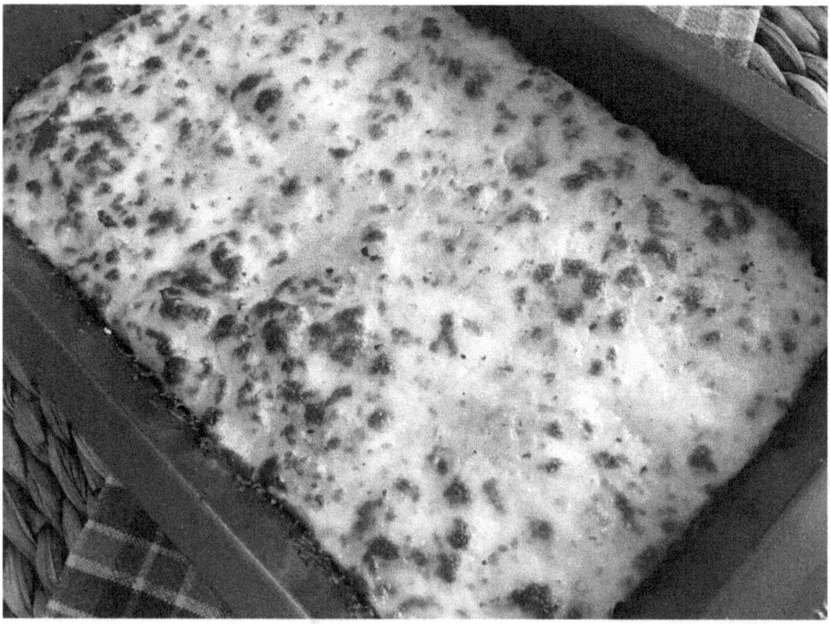

Cheesy Keto Breadsticks

This recipe takes about 33 minutes to prepare and makes 8 servings. There are two sets of directions for these, one for the bread dough and one for the cheesy top.

- Calories: 420
- Carbs: 5 grams
- Fat: 32 grams
- Fiber: 3 grams
- Protein: 29 grams

What to Use for the Cheesy Top

- 0.50 tsp of Italian seasoning
- 0.25 cups of parmesan cheese (shredded)
- 2 cups of mozzarella cheese (shredded)

What to Use for the Dough

- 0.50 cups of parmesan cheese (shredded)
- 1.75 cups of mozzarella cheese (shredded)
- 0.50 tsp of garlic powder
- 1 tsp of Italian seasoning
- 0.25 tsp of baking powder
- 0.25 tsp of salt
- 4 medium eggs

- 0.125 cups of cream cheese
- 0.75 cups of coconut flour
- 4.50 Tbsp of butter

Baking Instructions

- Preheat oven to 400F. Go grab a rectangle baking pan and grease it up while the oven is warming. Also, be sure to melt the butter, but cool it off in the fridge for 5 minutes.
- Grab a medium bowl and place inside it all the ingredients for the cheesy top (0.50 tsp of Italian seasoning, 0.25 cups of parmesan, and 2 cups of mozzarella). Set it to the side for later use.
- Grab a large bowl and place inside it the butter, cream cheese, salt, and eggs. Whisk everything together well.
- Add the baking powder, coconut flour, Italian seasoning, and garlic powder. Stir everything together until it combines well.
- Stir in the mozzarella (1.75 cups) and the parmesan 0.50 cups).
- Pour the dough batter into the baking pan.
- Use the seasoning and cheeses from the *Cheesy Top* ingredients to sprinkle on the dough.
- Bake for 10 minutes on the bottom or middle rack. Then take it out of the oven and use a pizza cutter to cut the dough vertically and horizontally to give it that breadstick shape.

- Bake for another 15 minutes.
- Move the bread sticks to the top rack and bake for another 2 minutes, so the cheesy top melts and browns correctly.

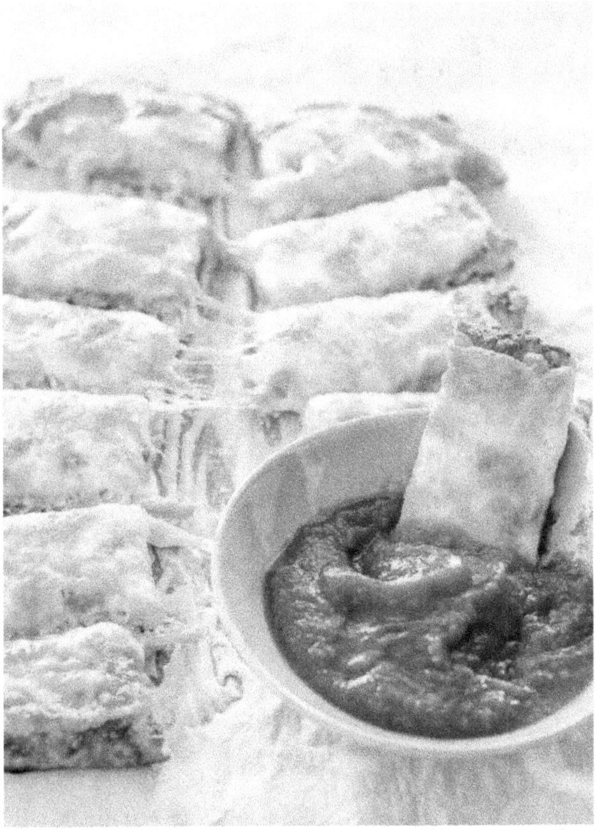

Cheese and Cauliflower Breadsticks

This recipe takes about 50 minutes to prepare and bake and makes 8 servings.

Mozzarella will pop up twice in this recipe. Once for the dough and another for the cheesy topping. Both of them should be shredded.

- Calories: 174
- Carbs: 4 grams
- Fat: 11 grams
- Fiber: 1 gram
- Protein: 13 grams

What to Use

- 1 cup of mozzarella cheese (shredded, for the topping to use near the end)
- 2 cups of mozzarella (shredded, for the dough)
- 1 tsp of salt
- 1 tsp of pepper
- 4 cloves of garlic (minced)
- 3 tsp of oregano
- 4 eggs
- 4 cups of cauliflower (riced)

Baking Instructions

- Preheat to 425F. While that is warming up grab a baking sheet and line it with parchment paper.

- Heat up the riced cauliflower in the microwave and heat it up for 10 minutes. Let it cool down (no more steam should be rising off of it).

- Grab a large bowl and place inside it the pepper, salt, garlic, oregano, eggs, and mozzarella (2 cups), and cauliflower.

- Separate the dough into 2 halves and shape both of them into rectangles.

- Bake for 25 minutes.

- Stop baking them and take them out of the oven so you can use a pizza cutter to cut them vertically and horizontally, creating a breadstick shape. Use the mozzarella (1 cup) to sprinkle on top.

- Bake for another 5 minutes.

Keto Crazy Breadsticks

This recipe takes about 25 minutes to prepare and bake and makes 6 servings. There are two sets of ingredients listed here. One for the dough and the other for the topping.

- Calories: 425
- Carbs: 10 grams
- Fat: 34 grams
- Fiber: 4 grams
- Protein: 24 grams

What to Use for the Dough

- 0.25 cups of butter (melted)
- 2 large eggs
- 1.50 cups of mozzarella (shredded)
- 0.50 tsp of xanthan gum
- 0.50 tsp of salt
- 0.50 tsp of garlic powder
- 2 tsp of baking powder
- 0.3125 cups of coconut flour
- 1 cup of almond flour

What to Use for the Topping

- 0.50 tsp of garlic powder

- 2 Tbsp of parmesan cheese
- 3 Tbsp of butter

Baking Instructions

- Preheat oven to 400F. While that is warming up go and grab a baking tray and line it up with parchment paper.
- Grab a large bowl and place inside it the xanthan gum, salt, garlic powder, baking powder, coconut flour, and almond flour. Whisk it all together.
- In a second large (microwave safe) bowl melt the mozzarella in a microwave for 2 minutes.
- Add the eggs and butter into the mozzarella.
- Add the contents from the fist bowl (the coconut flour, almond flour, and all their buddies) into the bowl of mozzarella, eggs, and butter. Stir everything together until it combines well.
- Place the dough onto the baking tray and roll it into a flat circle with a rolling pin.
- Use a pizza cutter to slice the dough horizontally and vertically to create stick like shapes.
- Mix together the topping ingredients: the garlic powder, parmesan cheese, and butter. Sprinkle them atop the dough.
- Bake for 15 minutes.

Easy Keto Sesame Breadsticks

This recipe takes 25 minutes to bake and prepare and makes 5 servings.

- Calories: 246
- Carbs: 4 grams
- Fat: 17 grams
- Fiber: 3 grams
- Protein: 14 grams

What to Use

- 1 Tbsp of olive oil
- 0.25 cups of almond flour
- 0.50 tsp of sesame seeds
- 1 tsp of pink Himalayan salt
- 1 medium egg white

Baking Instructions

- Preheat oven to 320F. While that is warming up go and get a baking tray and line it with parchment paper.
- Grab a large bowl and whisk the egg white. Then add the Himalayan salt, almond flour, and olive oil. Only use half of the olive oil (0.50 Tbsp). Do the same with the salt, only adding half (0.50 tsp) Save the rest of the olive oil and salt for later use.

- Stir and mix everything until they begin to combine.
- Use your hands to knead the dough. You are aiming for the dough to be soft but not overly sticky. If you run into trouble here and it does become too sticky, add some lukewarm water to loosen it up.
- Smear the rest of the salt and olive oil over the baking tray with parchment paper. Spread the sesame seeds there as well.
- Divide the dough into five pieces. Roll them into the shape of breadsticks.
- Place the breadsticks onto the baking tray and roll them all over the olive oil, salt, and sesame seeds.
- Bake for 20 minutes.

Keto Bread Twists

This recipe takes about 26 minutes to prepare and bake and makes 10 servings.

- Calories: 200
- Carbs: 20 grams
- Fat: 18 grams
- Fiber: 6 grams
- Protein: 15 grams

What to Use

- 2 medium egg (one of them is for egg wash)
- 0.25 cups of green pesto
- 0.375 cups of butter
- 1.50 cups of mozzarella (shredded)
- 1 tsp of baking powder
- 0.50 tsp of salt
- 4 Tbsp of coconut flour
- 0.25 cups of almond flour

Baking Instructions

- Preheat oven to 350F. While that is warming up get a baking sheet and line it with parchment paper. Also, take one of the eggs and whisk it to make the egg wash, then set aside for later.

- Get a large bowl and place inside it the almond flour, coconut flour, salt, and baking powder.
- Grab a large bowl (microwave safe) and place inside it the butter and mozzarella cheese. Melt them together in the microwave for 1 minute. Stir them together.
- Add 1 egg to the cheese and butter. Stir it until it blends together.
- Transfer the almond flour, coconut flour, salt, and baking powder into the butter, cheese, and egg mixture. Stir together until the dough takes form.
- Transfer the dough onto the baking sheet. Roll it into a rectangular shape with a rolling pin.
- Take the pesto and sprinkle it onto the dough.
- Cut the dough, using a pizza cutter, into one-inch strips. Twist the dough using your hands.
- Brush the bread twists with the egg wash.
- Bake for 20 minutes.

Cheesy Keto Garlic Bread

This recipe takes about 25 minutes to prepare and makes 10 servings.

This is not technically a breadstick, but this chapter is as good as any other placement for it. If desired, you can cut the dough into a breadstick shape but doing so will affect the serving size.

- Calories: 117
- Carbs: 3 grams
- Fat: 10 grams
- Fiber: 1 grams
- Protein: 6 grams

What to Use

- 1 medium egg
- 0.25 tsp of salt
- 1 tsp of baking powder
- 1 Tbsp of parsley (dried)
- 1 Tbsp of garlic (crushed)
- 2 Tbsp of cream cheese
- 0.75 cups of almond flour
- 0.50 cups of mozzarella cheese (shredded)

Baking Instructions

- Preheat oven to 425F. While that is warming up go and grab a baking tray.
- Grab a large (microwave safe) bowl and place inside it the mozzarella cheese, almond flour, cream cheese, baking powder, and salt.
- Gently stir the mixture till it blends well.
- Microwave for 30 seconds.
- Add the egg into the bowl and stir it till it blends.
- Transfer the dough onto the baking tray. Make sure to mold it into the shape of garlic bread. Cut the dough with a pizza cutter.
- Sprinkle the parsley atop the garlic bread dough.
- Bake for 15 minutes.

Fathead Rosemary Garlic Flatbread

This recipe takes about 25 minutes to prepare and makes 4 servings.

If desired, you can cut the dough into a breadstick shape but doing so will affect the serving size. This is a fathead dough recipe, and as such, know that you will be using your hands, the dough will be sticky, and things will get messy.

- Calories: 176
- Carbs: 3 grams
- Fat: 15 grams
- Fiber: 0.7 grams
- Protein: 8 grams

What to Use

- 2 cloves of garlic (crushed)
- 0.50 tsp of rosemary
- 2 tbsp of butter
- 2 Tbsp of coconut flour
- 1 medium egg
- 0.0625 cups of cream cheese
- 1 cup of mozzarella cheese

Baking Instructions

- Preheat oven to 400F. While that is warming up grab a cookie sheet and grease it up.

- Grab a medium (microwave safe) bowl and place inside it the cream cheese and mozzarella. Heat it up for 1 minute. Stir the cheese until it combines well.

- Add the egg (make sure it is beaten first) and the coconut flour. Stir them until they combine together well.

- Use your hands to spread the dough onto the cookie sheet.

- In a separate bowl, combine the butter, garlic, and rosemary. Mix them up and then use it to brush over the bread.

- Bake for 15 minutes.

Chapter 10: All The Rest

If all the different types of recipes for bread replacements were not enough for you, then consider this chapter a little extra. Some of these do veer away from what people think of when they hear the word "bread" but give them all a little perusal anyway. You just may be very surprised with what you see.

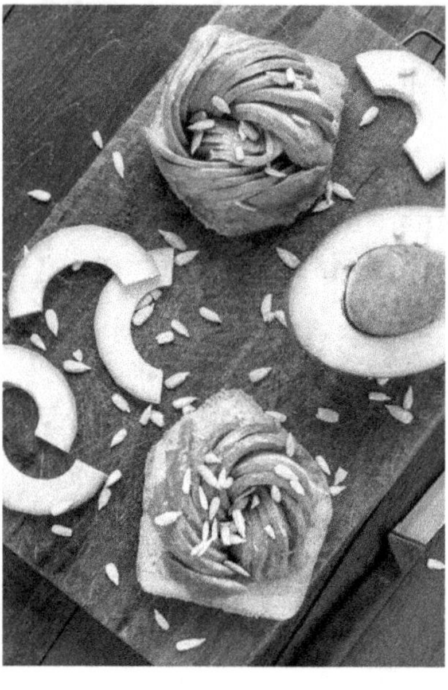

Keto Avocado Toast

This recipe takes about 40 minutes to prepare and bake and makes 12 servings.

Two sets of instructions and ingredients are listed here. One for the bread dough. The other for the avocado topping.

- Calories: 350
- Carbs: 6 grams
- Fat: 32 grams
- Fiber: 10 grams
- Protein: 5 grams

What to Use for the Avocado Topping

- 0.25 tsp of sea salt
- 2 Tbsp of sunflower seeds
- 1 medium avocado

What to Use for the Dough

- 0.50 tsp of sea salt
- 0.50 tsp of xanthan gum
- 2 cups of almond flour
- 1 tsp of baking soda
- 7 large eggs
- 2 Tbsp of coconut oil

- 0.50 cups of butter (melted)

Baking Instructions for the Dough

- Preheat oven to 350F. While that is warming up melt the butter (using a large microwave-safe bowl) in the microwave for 1 minute. Also, make sure to grab a baking pan and line it with parchment paper.

- Beat the eggs for 2 minutes with an electric mixer. May take longer without an electric mixer.

- Add the coconut oil and butter to the bowl of eggs. The butter should be cooled down a bit after melting. Beat everything together until it combines well

- Add the baking soda, almond flour, xanthan gum, and sea salt to the bowl of eggs. Stir them till they mix well.

- Transfer the batter into the pan.

- Bake for 45 minutes.

Instructions for the Avocado Topping

- Cut your avocado in half and make sure to remove the pit. Carefully peel away the shell.

- Slice the entire avocado into thin slices.

- Gently push and press the slices of avocado until they become long strips.

- Roll the strips into spiraled, hooked, shapes.

- Use the sunflower seeds and sea salt to sprinkle atop the avocado.

- Place the avocado topping on the toast. The toast should be cooled off enough but still hot enough to enjoy it to its fullest.

Keto Pizza Crust

This recipe takes about 20 minutes to prepare and bake and makes 1 pizza crust (or 8 slices of pizza).

- Calories: 110
- Carbs: 5 grams
- Fat: 7 grams
- Fiber: 3 grams
- Protein: 9 grams

What to Use

- 0.75 cups of coconut flour
- 2 large eggs
- 2 Tbsp of cream cheese (cubed)
- 1.50 cups of mozzarella (shredded)

Baking Instructions

- Preheat oven to 425F. While that is warming up go and grab a pizza pan (or any baking tray) and line it with parchment paper.
- Grab a large bowl and place inside it both the mozzarella and cream cheese. Place it in the microwave and heat up for 60 seconds. Stir it till it blends, then heat up for another 60 seconds. Stir it again.

- Beat the eggs. When that is done stir the beaten eggs and coconut flour together. Mix them together until they blend well

- Combine the mozzarella, cream cheese, eggs, and coconut flour together.

- Knead them with your hands until it molds together into a dough. If it starts to harden, then microwave it for another 15 seconds.

- Spread the dough onto the pan. Roll it till it flattens with a rolling pin. Poke some holes in the dough before baking.

- Bake for 6 minutes. Stop the baking so you can poke some more holes into the forming crust, then bake again for another 7 minutes.

Keto Cauliflower Pizza Crust

This recipe takes about 60 minutes to prepare and bake and makes 1 pizza crust (or 8 slices of pizza).

- Calories: 59
- Carbs: 4 grams
- Fat: 4 grams
- Fiber: 1 gram
- Protein: 5 grams

What to Use

- 0.25 tsp of salt
- 0.25 tsp of black ground pepper
- 1 tsp of garlic (chopped)
- 1 medium egg
- 0.25 cups of parsley (chopped)
- 0.50 cups of blended Italian cheeses
- 1 cup of water (boiling)
- Half a head of cauliflower (chopped up)

Baking Instructions

- Start boiling some water.
- Make sure to chop up the cauliflower. Also, chop up the parsley.

- Place the boiling water in a saucepan. Place the chopped cauliflower into the boiling water and cover it. This is to steam the cauliflower. Let the cauliflower steam for 15 minutes.

- When ready, go grab a large bowl and place the cauliflower inside it. Be careful here, as the cauliflower was sitting in boiling water, don't burn yourself. Stir the cauliflower gradually.

- Place the bowl of steamed cauliflower in the refrigerator to cool off for 15 minutes.

- Preheat over to 450F. While that is warming up go and grab a pizza pan (or any baking tray) and place parchment paper on top of it.

- Take the bowl of cauliflower out of the fridge. Add the pepper, salt, garlic, egg, parsley, and blended Italian cheese to the bowl. Stir until they mix together well.

- Pour the cauliflower dough mixture onto the pizza pan.

- Use a rolling pin to flatten the cauliflower dough and shape it into a pizza crust. Poke some holes into the dough before baking.

- Bake for 15 minutes.

Keto English Muffins

This recipe takes about 15 minutes to prepare and bake and makes 3 servings.

- Calories: 159
- Carbs: 20 grams
- Fat: 15 grams
- Fiber: 9 grams
- Protein: 12 grams

What to Use

- 3 Tbsp of butter
- 0.25 tsp of salt
- 0.50 tsp baking powder
- 2 Tbsp coconut flour
- 2 eggs

Baking Instructions

- Grab a large bowl and place inside it the salt, coconut flour, and baking soda.
- Take the eggs and add them into the bowl. Whisk so everything combines. Let is settle for 3 minutes.
- Turn the stove top on medium-high. Let the butter melt in a frying pan, then add three separate dollops of the batter into the pan.

- Let them fry for 3 minutes. Then flip them over and fry the opposite side for another three minutes.
- Alternatively, if you would like you can bake them in the oven for 10 minutes. Doing so may make the finished product seem more like buns then English muffins and will also lower the fat count.

Keto Pancakes

This recipe takes about 20 minutes to prepare and bake and makes 2 servings.

There are two sets of ingredients and instructions listed. One for the pancakes, and another for the toppings. However, there is not much preparation at all for the toppings.

- Calories: 425
- Carbs: 40 grams
- Fat: 40 grams
- Fiber: 3 grams
- Protein: 13 grams

What to Use for the Pancakes

- 0.25 cup of coconut oil
- 1 Tbsp of psyllium husk powder
- 0.875 cups of cottage cheese
- 4 medium eggs

What to Use for the Toppings

- 0.25 tsp of blueberries. Raspberries or strawberries would also work fine. Remember that no matter what you use, fresh is the best. 0.25 tsp is only approximate, a handful is all you will really need.
- 1 cup of heavy whipping cream.

Baking Instructions

- Grab a medium bowl and place inside it the psyllium husk powder, cottage cheese, and eggs. Stir and mix everything together. Let it sit for 8 minutes so it can thicken.

- Turn the stovetop on low-medium and heat up the butter in a skillet.

- Place the pancake mix in the skillet. Fry them for 4 minutes. Then flip and fry the opposite side for another 4 minutes.

- Whip the heavy whipping cream in a separate bowl until it softens.

- Top the pancakes with the whipped cream and the blueberries.

Keto Blueberry Almond Brownies

This recipe takes about 50 minutes to prepare and bake and makes 20 servings.

This recipe contains stevia, but any non-sugar-based sweetener will work.

- Calories: 199
- Carbs: 5 grams
- Fat: 18 grams
- Fiber: 3 grams
- Protein: 5 grams

What to Use

- 0.125 cups of blueberries
- 0.25 tsp of salt
- 2 large eggs
- 8 Tbsp of butter (melted)
- 1 cup of cream cheese (melted)
- 2 cups of stevia
- 0.25 tsp of vanilla extract
- 0.50 tsp of baking powder
- 0.50 cups of flaxseed meal
- 3 cups of almond meal

Baking Instructions

- Preheat oven to 350F. While that is warming up grab a cake baking pan and place parchment paper over it.

- Go get a large bowl and place inside it the almond meal, flaxseed meal, baking powder, vanilla extract, cream cheese, stevia, butter, and salt. Mix everything together.

- Transfer all of the contents into the baking pan and smooth out the top until it is even.

- Place the blueberries atop the batter.

- Bake for 30 minutes. Let cool for 15 minutes.

Low Carb Cloud Bread French Toast

This recipe takes about 10 minutes to prepare and bake and makes 4 servings.

This recipe contains stevia, but any non-sugar-based sweetener would work. You can use more pieces of bread to make the French Toast if you like, but that will throw off the serving count and nutritional data.

- Calories: 283
- Carbs: 3 grams
- Fat: 20 grams
- Fiber: 1 gram
- Protein: 18 grams

What to Use

- 0.125 cups of butter
- 0.25 tsp of salt
- 0.50 tsp of vanilla extract
- 1 tsp of cinnamon (ground)
- 0.25 tsp of stevia
- 0.25 cups of heavy cream
- 2 medium eggs
- 2-8 slices of a low carb bread (use one of the recipes listed in this book for these slices. The Keto Cloud Bread Buns would work nicely).

Baking Instructions

- Grab a large bowl and place inside it the salt, vanilla, cinnamon, stevia, heavy cream, and eggs. Whisk everything together until they blend well.

- Put 2 pieces of the bread slices and let it soak for 1 minute. After the minute passes, flip it over and soak the other side. Repeat this step for how many ever pieces of French Toast you plan on making.

- Turn the stove top on medium-high and get out a skillet. Melt the butter in the pan.

- Place the soaked bread into the skillet. You should be able to fit 4 pieces at a time.

- Cook the bread for 3 minutes. Then flip over and heat the opposite side.

- If desired, repeat the previous step for however many pieces of French Toast you plan on making.

Flaxseed Crispy Keto Waffles

This recipe takes about 10 minutes to prepare and bake and makes 4 servings.

- Calories: 500
- Carbs: 19 grams
- Fat: 42 grams
- Fiber: 16 grams
- Protein: 18 grams

What to Use

- 2 tsp of cinnamon (ground)
- 0.75 cups of avocado oil
- 0.50 cups of water
- 5 large eggs
- 1 tsp of salt
- 1 Tbsp of baking powder
- 2 cups of golden flaxseed (grounded)

Baking Instructions

- Get a waffle maker and turn it on to the medium setting.
- Grab a large bowl and place inside it the baking powder and flaxseed. Whisk them together until they combine well.

- Grab a blender and place inside it the water, avocado oil, and eggs. Blend on high for 30 seconds.

- Transfer the contents from the blender into the bowl of flaxseed and baking powder. Stir them together until they blend well. Then let it sit and settle for 3 minutes.

- When ready, add the cinnamon into the mixture. Stir it until it mixes with everything else.

- Separate the batter into 4 and place each of the pieces onto the waffle maker. Do so one at a time. Cook each one separately until the waffle maker tells you it's done.

Keto No Bake Peanut Butter Cookies

This recipe takes about 55 minutes to prepare and bake and makes 20 servings.

Alright, to be clear there is chocolate in this recipe, and it is the only thing in this book you will find that contains chocolate. However, there are chocolate chip baking options out there that do not contain any sugar. One recommendation is *Lilly's Dark Chocolate.* It can be purchased through Amazon. Or if you know of another non-sugar-based chocolate chip, that can be used as well. Stevia is also in this recipe, but any non-sugar-based sweetener will work. Another warning, your hands will probably get dirty.

- Calories: 99
- Carbs: 4 grams
- Fat: 7 grams
- Fiber: 3 grams
- Protein: 4 grams

What to Use

- 2 cups of chocolate chips (that do not contain any sugar, see notes above.)
- 5 Tbsp of stevia.
- 2 cups of peanut butter (smooth peanut butter is recommended for this recipe)
- 0.75 cups of almond flour

Non-Baking Instructions

- Go grab a baking tray and place parchment paper on top of it.

- Then go grab a large (microwave safe) bowl and place inside of it the stevia and peanut butter. Melt them for about 1 minute. Take them out and stir them together a bit.

- Put the coconut flour into the peanut butter and stir them until the batter starts to thicken up nice and well.

- Use your hands to mold four separate small balls.

- Place the molded balls of peanut butter on the baking tray. Use a fork or knife to flatten them down, so they resemble cookies.

- Freeze them for 20 minutes.

- When ready, take them out of the freezer.

- Melt the chocolate chips in a small (microwave safe) bowl.

- Take each cookie and individually dip them into the melted chocolate. If having trouble pulling this step off, try using two forks to pincer the cookies. Make sure that each cookie is completely covered with the chocolate.

- Place the cookies in the fridge for about 30 minutes, or until they firm up.

Lemon Keto Danish Pastries

This recipe takes about 25 minutes to prepare and bake and makes 6 servings.

There are two sets of ingredients and instructions listed for this recipe. One is for the filling, the other is for the pastry.

- Calories: 349
- Carbs: 8 grams
- Fat: 31 grams
- Fiber: 3 grams
- Protein: 9 grams

What to Use for the Filling

- 1 zest of lemon
- 0.50 tsp of lemon extract
- 3 Tbsp of stevia
- 1 cup of cream cheese

What to Use for the Pastry

- 1 Tbsp of vanilla extract
- 4.50 tsp of butter
- 1.50 cups of mozzarella (shredded)
- 2 large eggs
- 1.25 tsp of baking powder

- 1 Tbsp of stevia
- 0.25 cups of coconut flour
- 0.75 cups of almond flour

Baking Instructions for the Filling

- Grab a medium bowl and place inside it the zest of lemon, lemon extract, stevia, and cream cheese. An electric hand mixer is recommended here for the mixing. A low speed is also recommended. Mix until everything combines well. After it starts to combine, turn the speed on the mixer to high and continue to mix until the blend gives off a fluffy appearance. Set the bowl off to the side so you can use it later.

Baking Instructions for the Pastry

- Preheat oven to 350F. While that is warming up go and grab a cookie sheet and place parchment paper on it.
- Grab a large mixing bowl and place inside it the baking powder, stevia, coconut flour, and almond flour. Whisk everything together until it combines well.
- Grab another small bowl and place one of the eggs inside it, and also put the vanilla extract inside it. Whisk them together.
- Pour the egg and vanilla extract into the bowl of almond flour, coconut flour, and all their friends. Mix them together until they blend. The egg should not disappear and entirely mix in. The yolk should remain visible.

- Take the second egg and place that in a separate small bowl. Whisk it and set aside for later. This will be used for your egg wash.

- Place both the butter and mozzarella in a (microwave safe) medium bowl and heat it up for 1 minute. Stir it up and then microwave it for another 30 seconds (keep in mind that microwaves vary so adjust accordingly).

- Place the melted butter and mozzarella into the bowl of eggs, almond flour, and all their friends.

- Use your hand to knead the dough until it takes proper form. Try to mold it into the shape of a disk. Then use a rolling pin to flatten and form it into a rectangle shape.

- Cut the dough into 12 separate rectangular pieces.

- Transfer the filling onto the pastry dough. Place it upon each one separately.

- Take the pieces that do not have filling on them and place them on top of the pieces that do have a filling (sandwich them together). Close then pinch the edges together and use a fork to press them together.

- Place tiny holes into each of the pastries. This will help the steam exit them properly.

- Use the egg wash to brush the pastries.

- Bake for 18 minutes. These pastries can burn up fast, so keep an eye on them as they are baking.

Keto Low Carb Vanilla Almond Yellow Butter Cake

This recipe takes about 40 minutes to prepare and bake and makes 8 servings.

That's right, we snuck a cake in.

- Calories: 187
- Carbs: 6 grams
- Fat: 18 grams
- Fiber: 2 grams
- Protein: 8 grams

What to Use

- 0.25 tsp of salt
- 1 tsp of baking soda
- 2 Tbsp of tapioca flour
- 0.125 cups of flaxseed meal (golden)
- 1 cup of almond flour
- 0.25 tsp of stevia
- 0.50 tsp of almond extract (pure is the best)
- 1.50 tsp of vanilla extract
- 2 large eggs
- 4 tsp of erythritol

- 0.125 cups of butter

Baking Instructions

- Preheat oven to 350F. While that is warming up go and grab a loaf pan and place parchment paper over it. Also, grease up the pan (for baking this cake coconut oil is recommended to slick the pan).

- Grab a medium bowl and place inside it the butter and erythritol. Beat them until they cream together.

- Add the stevia, almond extract, vanilla extract, and eggs into the bowl of butter and erythritol. Whisk everything together until they blend well.

- Grab a separate medium bowl and place inside it the baking powder, tapioca flour, flaxseed meal, and almond flour. Whisk everything together until it blends together well.

- Transfer the bowl of tapioca flour and all his friends into the bowl of eggs, erythritol and all of their buddies. Whisk everything together until it combines well.

- Transfer the batter into the baking pan. Spread it out to even the top and fill the pan.

- Bake for 30 minutes. Let cool for 5.

Keto Mozzarella Sticks

This recipe takes about 50 minutes to prepare and bake and makes 10 servings.

- Calories: 390
- Carbs: 3 grams
- Fat: 3 grams
- Fiber: 1 gram
- Protein: 35 grams

What to Use

- 0.25 tsp of salt
- 0.25 tsp of black pepper
- 1 medium egg
- 1 tsp of Italian seasoning
- 0.50 tsp of garlic powder
- 1 tsp of baking powder
- 0.125 cups of coconut flour
- 0.50 cups of parmesan cheese
- 4 sticks of mozzarella string cheese (one ounce each)

Baking Instructions

- Grab a small bowl and place inside it the pepper, salt, and egg. Whisk everything together.

- Grab a medium bowl and place inside it the parmesan cheese, coconut flour, baking powder, garlic powder, and Italian seasoning.
- Get the cheese sticks ready and dip each on separately into the bowl of egg, pepper, and salt.
- Roll the cheese sticks in the bowl of parmesan and all his friends.
- Repeat the previous two steps again. A double coating of the cheese is recommended for this recipe.
- Put the cheese sticks in a container and leave them in the freezer to chill for 25 minutes.
- Turn the stove top on and get a pan for frying ready. Use olive oil to get the pan nice and slicked up.
- Fry the cheese sticks for 90 seconds on each side. If there is any excess oil, drain it with a paper towel.

Conclusion

Thanks for making it through to the end of *Ketogenic Bread: Low Carb Recipes for Ketogenic Bread, Buns, Crackers, and More!* Let's hope it was informative and able to provide you with all of the tools you need to achieve your goals whatever they may be.

The next step is to put all of your new knowledge to use and start making the transformation into the keto lifestyle. Head on down to the supermarket, your local health food store, or go looking online for the proper ingredients and get ready to leave the carbs and sugars in the past. By downloading this book, you have taken a serious and important step in starting to retrain your body to select a better resource and getting those ketones to turn you into a fat-burning machine. The positive change that you have been looking for begins as soon as you start putting all you have learned to use. The waiting is over.

As with everything else in life, you do have to put in the work to reach the results that you want, and as we all know, dieting or changing habits (eating and otherwise), is going to be a long-term commitment. When you get to see the changes in your body and feel the mental clarity and bursts of energy that go along with making the move to keto, you will know that the commitment was absolutely worth it.

Are You a Helpful Person?

I have put my heart and soul in this book, and it took me a lot of time & research to finish it. If you found this book useful, please consider leaving a review on Amazon. It will be such a nice thing for you to do, not only for me, but for other readers just like you. Although I know it's time consuming, a good review can make my day, and I read all of them ☺

That's it! If you'd like to ask me about the recipes, the ketogenic diet, or anything else you'd like to ask.

Best regards,
Timothy Turner

www.ingramcontent.com/pod-product-compliance
Lightning Source LLC
Chambersburg PA
CBHW071255220526
45468CB00001B/129
9781723369797